Menopause marks a significant transition in a woman's life, bringing with it a host of physical and emotional changes. For many, this period can be challenging, with symptoms such as weight gain, hot flashes, mood swings, and decreased energy. The Galveston Diet, designed specifically to address the unique needs of women going through menopause, offers a comprehensive approach to manage these symptoms through nutrition and lifestyle changes.

"The Galveston Diet Cookbook to Manage Menopause: 100+ Nutrient-Rich Recipes to Support Your Journey" is your essential guide to navigating menopause with vitality and wellness. This cookbook is more than just a collection of recipes; it is a holistic resource designed to empower women to take control of their health and well-being during this pivotal stage of life.

The Galveston Diet focuses on anti-inflammatory and low-carbohydrate foods that are rich in essential nutrients, tailored to support hormonal balance and overall health. By incorporating these principles into your daily routine, you can alleviate menopause symptoms, boost your energy levels, and maintain a healthy weight.

Within these pages, you'll find over 100 delicious and easy-to-make recipes that cater to every meal of the day, from wholesome breakfasts and satisfying lunches to delectable dinners and guilt-free desserts. Each recipe is crafted to provide the right balance of proteins, healthy fats, and fiber, ensuring you get the most out of every bite.

In addition to the recipes, this cookbook offers practical tips and insights on meal planning, grocery shopping, and cooking techniques, making it easier than ever to embrace the Galveston Diet lifestyle. Whether you're new to the Galveston Diet or looking to expand your culinary repertoire, this cookbook is your companion for a healthier, happier menopause journey.

Embark on this journey with us and discover how the right nutrition can transform your menopause experience, bringing you renewed energy, balanced hormones, and a greater sense of well-being. Welcome to **"The Galveston Diet Cookbook to Manage Menopause"** – your guide to thriving through menopause and beyond.

1. Grilled Salmon with Lemon and Dill

Ingredients:

• 4 salmon fillets (about 4•6 oz each)
• 2 tbsp olive oil
• 2 tbsp fresh lemon juice
• 2 tsp dried dill weed
• 1 tsp garlic powder
• Salt and pepper to taste

Instructions:

1. Preheat grill to medium•high heat.

2. In a small bowl, whisk together the olive oil, lemon juice, dill, and garlic powder. Season with salt and pepper.

3. Place the salmon fillets on a large piece of foil. Brush the salmon with the lemon•dill mixture, making sure to coat the top and sides.

4. Grill the salmon for 12•15 minutes, flipping halfway through, or until the fish flakes easily with a fork and is cooked through.

5. Serve the grilled salmon immediately, garnished with additional lemon slices and fresh dill if desired.

This recipe is a great option for the Galveston Diet, as it features heart•healthy salmon, anti•inflammatory lemon and dill, and is grilled rather than fried. The Galveston Diet emphasizes lean proteins, healthy fats, and anti•inflammatory foods to help manage menopausal symptoms.

2. Chicken Caesar Salad

Ingredients:

• 4 boneless, skinless chicken breasts
• 1 tbsp olive oil
• 1 tsp garlic powder
• Salt and pepper to taste
• 6 cups chopped romaine lettuce
• 1/4 cup grated Parmesan cheese
• 2 tbsp lemon juice
• 2 tbsp olive oil
• 1 tsp Dijon mustard
• 1 garlic clove, minced
• Salt and pepper to taste

Instructions:

1. Preheat grill or grill pan to medium•high heat.

2. Rub the chicken breasts with 1 tbsp olive oil and season with garlic powder, salt, and pepper.

3. Grill the chicken for 5•7 minutes per side, or until cooked through. Allow to cool slightly, then slice or shred the chicken.

4. In a large salad bowl, combine the chopped romaine lettuce, grilled chicken, and Parmesan cheese.

5. In a small bowl, whisk together the lemon juice, 2 tbsp olive oil, Dijon mustard, minced garlic, salt, and pepper to make the dressing.

6. Drizzle the dressing over the salad and toss to coat.

7. Serve immediately.

This Chicken Caesar Salad is a great option for the Galveston Diet, as it features lean protein from the grilled chicken, healthy fats from the olive oil and Parmesan, and anti•inflammatory ingredients like lemon and garlic. The Galveston Diet emphasizes these types of nutrient•dense, anti•inflammatory foods to help manage menopausal symptoms.

3. Quinoa and Black Bean Salad

Ingredients:

- 1 cup uncooked quinoa, rinsed
- 1 (15 oz) can black beans, rinsed and drained
- 1 cup diced cucumber
- 1 cup diced tomatoes
- 1/2 cup diced red onion
- 1/4 cup chopped fresh cilantro
- 2 tbsp olive oil
- 2 tbsp lime juice
- 1 tsp ground cumin
- 1/2 tsp garlic powder
- Salt and pepper to taste

Instructions:

1. Cook the quinoa according to package instructions. Allow to cool.

2. In a large bowl, combine the cooked quinoa, black beans, cucumber, tomatoes, red onion, and cilantro.

3. In a small bowl, whisk together the olive oil, lime juice, cumin, garlic powder, salt, and pepper.

4. Pour the dressing over the quinoa and bean mixture and toss to coat evenly.

5. Refrigerate for at least 30 minutes to allow the flavors to meld.

6. Serve chilled or at room temperature.

This Quinoa and Black Bean Salad is an excellent choice for the Galveston Diet, as it is packed with plant•based protein, fiber, and anti•inflammatory ingredients. Quinoa is a nutrient•dense whole grain, while black beans provide additional protein and fiber. The vegetables, herbs, and citrus dressing add antioxidants and anti•inflammatory properties to support menopausal health.

4. Shrimp Stir•Fry with Vegetables

Ingredients:

- 1 lb peeled and deveined shrimp
- 2 tbsp sesame oil
- 2 cloves garlic, minced
- 1 inch piece fresh ginger, peeled and grated
- 1 red bell pepper, sliced
- 1 cup broccoli florets
- 1 cup snow peas or snap peas
- 2 cups baby spinach
- 2 tbsp low•sodium soy sauce or coconut aminos
- 1 tbsp rice vinegar
- 1 tsp sesame seeds (optional)
- Salt and pepper to taste

Instructions:

1. Heat the sesame oil in a large skillet or wok over high heat.

2. Add the garlic and ginger and cook for 1 minute, stirring constantly, until fragrant.

3. Add the shrimp and stir•fry for 2•3 minutes until they start to turn pink.

4. Add the bell pepper, broccoli, and snow peas. Stir•fry for 3•4 minutes until the vegetables are crisp•tender.

5. Stir in the spinach and cook for 1 minute until wilted.

6. Add the soy sauce or coconut aminos and rice vinegar. Toss to coat everything evenly.

7. Remove from heat and sprinkle with sesame seeds, if using. Season with salt and pepper to taste.

8. Serve immediately over cauliflower rice or zucchini noodles.

This Shrimp Stir•Fry is a great option for the Galveston Diet, as it features lean protein from the shrimp, anti•inflammatory vegetables, and healthy fats from the sesame oil. The Galveston Diet emphasizes these types of nutrient•dense, anti•inflammatory foods to help manage menopausal symptoms.

5. Greek Yogurt Parfait with Berries

Ingredients:

• 2 cups plain Greek yogurt
• 1 cup mixed berries (such as blueberries, raspberries, and/or blackberries)
• 2 tbsp chopped walnuts or sliced almonds
• 1 tbsp honey (optional)

Instructions:

1. In a parfait glass or bowl, layer the Greek yogurt, berries, and nuts.

2. If desired, drizzle a small amount of honey over the top.

3. Repeat the layers until you reach the top of the glass or bowl.

4. Refrigerate until ready to serve.

This Greek Yogurt Parfait with Berries is an excellent choice for the Galveston Diet, as it provides a balance of protein, healthy fats, and antioxidants:

• Greek yogurt is a great source of protein and probiotics, which can help support gut health.
• Berries are packed with antioxidants and anti•inflammatory compounds.
• Nuts like walnuts and almonds provide healthy fats and additional fiber.
• Honey (if used) can provide a natural sweetener.

The Galveston Diet emphasizes nutrient•dense, anti•inflammatory foods like these to help manage menopausal symptoms. This parfait makes for a satisfying and nourishing breakfast, snack, or dessert.

6. Vegetable Frittata

Ingredients:

- 8 large eggs
- 1/4 cup unsweetened almond milk
- 1/4 cup grated Parmesan cheese
- 1 tsp dried oregano
- Salt and pepper to taste
- 1 tbsp olive oil
- 1 cup diced bell peppers
- 1 cup sliced mushrooms
- 1 cup chopped spinach
- 1/2 cup diced onion

Instructions:

1. Preheat your oven to 375°F.

2. In a large bowl, whisk together the eggs, almond milk, Parmesan cheese, oregano, salt, and pepper.

3. Heat the olive oil in a 9•inch oven•safe skillet over medium heat.

4. Add the bell peppers, mushrooms, spinach, and onion to the skillet. Sauté for 5•7 minutes, until the vegetables are tender.

5. Pour the egg mixture over the vegetables in the skillet, making sure the vegetables are evenly distributed.

6. Transfer the skillet to the preheated oven and bake for 18•22 minutes, or until the frittata is set and lightly golden on top.

7. Remove the frittata from the oven and let it cool for a few minutes before slicing and serving.

This Vegetable Frittata is an excellent choice for the Galveston Diet, as it is packed with nutrient•dense vegetables, protein•rich eggs, and healthy fats from the olive oil and Parmesan cheese. The Galveston Diet emphasizes these types of anti•inflammatory, nutrient•dense foods to help manage menopausal symptoms.

7. Lentil Soup

Ingredients:

- 1 tbsp olive oil
- 1 onion, diced
- 3 cloves garlic, minced
- 2 carrots, peeled and diced
- 2 celery stalks, diced
- 1 cup dried brown or green lentils, rinsed
- 4 cups low•sodium vegetable or chicken broth
- 1 (14.5 oz) can diced tomatoes
- 2 tsp dried thyme
- 1 tsp ground cumin
- Salt and pepper to taste
- 2 cups baby spinach or kale, chopped

Instructions:

1. In a large pot or Dutch oven, heat the olive oil over medium heat.

2. Add the onion, garlic, carrots, and celery. Sauté for 5•7 minutes, until the vegetables are softened.

3. Stir in the lentils, broth, diced tomatoes, thyme, and cumin. Season with salt and pepper.

4. Bring the soup to a boil, then reduce heat and simmer for 20•25 minutes, or until the lentils are tender.

5. Stir in the chopped spinach or kale and cook for an additional 2•3 minutes, until the greens are wilted.

6. Serve the lentil soup hot, garnished with additional herbs or a drizzle of olive oil if desired.

This Lentil Soup is an excellent choice for the Galveston Diet, as it is packed with plant•based protein, fiber, and anti•inflammatory ingredients. Lentils are a nutrient•dense legume, while the vegetables and herbs provide antioxidants and anti•inflammatory properties to support menopausal health.

8. Turkey Lettuce Wraps

Ingredients:

• 1 lb ground turkey
• 1 tbsp olive oil
• 1 onion, diced
• 2 cloves garlic, minced
• 1 tbsp grated fresh ginger
• 1 tbsp low•sodium soy sauce or coconut aminos
• 1 tsp sesame oil
• 1 tsp rice vinegar
• 1/4 tsp red pepper flakes (optional)
• Salt and pepper to taste
• 1 head of romaine or butter lettuce, leaves separated

Toppings (optional):
• Shredded carrots
• Sliced cucumber
• Chopped green onions
• Toasted sesame seeds

Instructions:

1. In a large skillet or wok, heat the olive oil over medium•high heat.

2. Add the ground turkey and cook, breaking it up with a wooden spoon, until browned and cooked through, about 5•7 minutes.

3. Add the onion, garlic, and ginger. Cook for 2•3 minutes, until fragrant.

4. Stir in the soy sauce or coconut aminos, sesame oil, rice vinegar, and red pepper flakes (if using). Season with salt and pepper. Spoon the turkey mixture into the lettuce leaves.

5. Top with desired toppings like shredded carrots, sliced cucumber, chopped green onions, and toasted sesame seeds. Serve immediately.

These Turkey Lettuce Wraps are a great option for the Galveston Diet, as they feature lean protein from the ground turkey, anti•inflammatory ingredients like ginger and garlic, and a light, refreshing presentation. The Galveston Diet emphasizes these types of nutrient•dense, anti•inflammatory foods to help manage menopausal symptoms.

9. Zucchini Noodles with Pesto

Ingredients:

- 3 medium zucchini, spiralized or julienned into noodles
- 2 cups fresh basil leaves
- 1/4 cup pine nuts or walnuts
- 2 cloves garlic
- 1/4 cup grated Parmesan cheese
- 2 tbsp olive oil
- 1 tbsp lemon juice
- Salt and pepper to taste

Instructions:

1. In a food processor or blender, combine the basil, pine nuts or walnuts, garlic, Parmesan, olive oil, and lemon juice. Pulse until a smooth pesto forms. Season with salt and pepper to taste.

2. In a large skillet or sauté pan, heat a small amount of olive oil over medium heat. Add the zucchini noodles and sauté for 2•3 minutes, just until they start to soften slightly. Be careful not to overcook.

3. Remove the zucchini noodles from the heat and toss with the prepared pesto until the noodles are evenly coated.

4. Serve the zucchini noodles with pesto immediately, garnished with additional Parmesan cheese, pine nuts, or fresh basil if desired.

This Zucchini Noodles with Pesto dish is an excellent choice for the Galveston Diet, as it features:

- Zucchini noodles, which are low in carbs and high in fiber and nutrients
- Basil•based pesto, which provides anti•inflammatory benefits
- Healthy fats from the olive oil and pine nuts/walnuts
- Parmesan cheese for added protein and flavor

The Galveston Diet emphasizes these types of nutrient•dense, anti•inflammatory foods to help manage menopausal symptoms.

10. Grilled Chicken with Avocado Salsa

Ingredients:

• 4 boneless, skinless chicken breasts
• 1 ripe avocado, diced
• 1/2 cup diced tomatoes
• 1/4 cup diced red onion
• 2 tbsp chopped fresh cilantro
• 1 tbsp lime juice
• 1 tsp olive oil
• Salt and pepper to taste

Instructions:

1. Preheat grill to medium•high heat.

2. Season the chicken breasts with salt and pepper.

3. Grill the chicken for 4•6 minutes per side, or until cooked through.

4. In a medium bowl, combine the diced avocado, tomatoes, red onion, cilantro, lime juice, and olive oil. Season with salt and pepper.

5. Serve the grilled chicken topped with the avocado salsa.

This dish is a great option for the Galveston Diet during menopause as it is high in healthy fats from the avocado, and the lean protein from the grilled chicken can help support muscle mass and bone health. The fresh vegetables and herbs also provide important nutrients and antioxidants. Remember to adjust portion sizes and side dishes as needed to fit your individual dietary needs during menopause.

11. Eggplant Parmesan

Ingredients:

- 2 medium eggplants, sliced into 1/2•inch thick rounds
- 1 cup whole wheat breadcrumbs
- 1/2 cup grated Parmesan cheese
- 2 eggs, beaten
- 2 cups marinara sauce
- 1 cup shredded part•skim mozzarella cheese

Instructions:

1. Preheat oven to 375°F. Lightly grease a baking sheet.

2. In a shallow bowl, combine the breadcrumbs and Parmesan cheese. In another shallow bowl, place the beaten eggs.

3. Dip the eggplant slices into the egg, then coat both sides with the breadcrumb mixture, pressing gently to adhere.

4. Arrange the breaded eggplant slices in a single layer on the prepared baking sheet.

5. Bake for 20•25 minutes, flipping halfway, until the eggplant is tender and the breading is golden brown.

6. Spread 1 cup of the marinara sauce in the bottom of a 9x13 inch baking dish. Arrange the baked eggplant slices in a single layer over the sauce.

7. Top the eggplant with the remaining 1 cup of marinara sauce and the shredded mozzarella cheese.

8. Bake for an additional 15•20 minutes, until the cheese is melted and bubbly.

9. Let stand for 5 minutes before serving.

This eggplant parmesan dish is a great option for the Galveston Diet during menopause as it is low in carbs, high in fiber, and provides a good source of plant•based protein and healthy fats. The eggplant and tomato•based sauce also provide important nutrients and antioxidants.

12. Cauliflower Rice Stir•Fry

Ingredients:

• 1 head of cauliflower, riced (about 4 cups riced cauliflower)
• 1 tbsp olive oil
• 1 clove garlic, minced
• 1 inch piece fresh ginger, grated
• 1 cup diced mixed vegetables (such as bell peppers, broccoli, snap peas)
• 2 tbsp low•sodium soy sauce or tamari
• 1 tsp sesame oil
• Salt and pepper to taste
• Chopped green onions and sesame seeds for garnish (optional)

Instructions:

1. To make the cauliflower rice, cut the cauliflower into florets and pulse in a food processor until it resembles rice•sized granules.

2. Heat the olive oil in a large skillet or wok over medium•high heat. Add the garlic and ginger and cook for 1 minute, until fragrant.

3. Add the riced cauliflower and mixed vegetables to the pan. Stir•fry for 5•7 minutes, until the cauliflower is tender•crisp.

4. Add the soy sauce and sesame oil. Toss to coat everything evenly.

5. Season with salt and pepper to taste.

6. Serve the cauliflower rice stir•fry warm, garnished with chopped green onions and sesame seeds if desired.

This cauliflower rice stir•fry is a great option for the Galveston Diet during menopause. Cauliflower is low in carbs and high in fiber, while the vegetables provide a variety of nutrients. The dish is also gluten•free and can be easily customized with your choice of protein, such as grilled chicken or tofu, to make it a complete meal.

13. Tuna Salad Stuffed Avocado

Ingredients:

- 2 (5 oz) cans of tuna, drained
- 2 tbsp mayonnaise (or Greek yogurt)
- 1 tbsp Dijon mustard
- 1 tbsp lemon juice
- 2 tbsp finely chopped celery
- 2 tbsp finely chopped red onion
- 2 tbsp chopped fresh parsley
- Salt and pepper to taste
- 2 ripe avocados, halved and pitted

Instructions:

1. In a medium bowl, combine the drained tuna, mayonnaise (or Greek yogurt), Dijon mustard, lemon juice, celery, red onion, and parsley. Mix well and season with salt and pepper to taste.

2. Scoop the tuna salad evenly into the 4 avocado halves.

3. Serve the tuna salad stuffed avocados immediately, or refrigerate until ready to serve.

This tuna salad stuffed avocado dish is an excellent option for the Galveston Diet during menopause. The avocado provides healthy fats, while the tuna is a lean protein source. The combination of the two is filling and nutritious. The added vegetables and herbs also provide important vitamins, minerals, and antioxidants.

This dish can be enjoyed as a light lunch or a satisfying snack. It's also easy to prepare and can be made ahead of time for a quick and convenient meal. Adjust the portion sizes as needed to fit your individual dietary needs during menopause.

14. Kale and Quinoa Salad

Ingredients:

- 1 cup cooked quinoa, cooled
- 4 cups chopped kale, stems removed
- 1 cup diced cucumber
- 1/2 cup diced red bell pepper
- 1/4 cup diced red onion
- 2 tbsp chopped fresh parsley
- 2 tbsp olive oil
- 2 tbsp lemon juice
- 1 tsp Dijon mustard
- 1 tsp honey
- Salt and pepper to taste

Instructions:

1. In a large bowl, combine the cooked quinoa, chopped kale, diced cucumber, red bell pepper, red onion, and parsley.

2. In a small bowl, whisk together the olive oil, lemon juice, Dijon mustard, and honey. Season with salt and pepper.

3. Pour the dressing over the kale and quinoa mixture and toss gently to coat everything evenly.

4. Let the salad sit for 5•10 minutes to allow the flavors to meld.

5. Serve the kale and quinoa salad chilled or at room temperature.

This kale and quinoa salad is an excellent choice for the Galveston Diet during menopause. Kale is a nutrient•dense leafy green that provides fiber, vitamins, and antioxidants. Quinoa is a gluten•free, high•protein grain that can help support muscle mass and bone health. The combination of vegetables, healthy fats from the olive oil, and the tangy dressing make this a well•balanced and satisfying meal.

You can adjust the portion sizes and add additional protein, such as grilled chicken or roasted chickpeas, to make this salad a complete and filling meal. This dish can also be prepared in advance and stored in the refrigerator for a quick and easy lunch or dinner option.

15. Baked Cod with Roasted Vegetables

Ingredients:

• 4 (6 oz) cod fillets
• 2 tbsp olive oil
• 1 lb mixed vegetables (such as broccoli, cauliflower, Brussels sprouts, carrots), cut into bite•sized pieces
• 1 red onion, sliced
• 2 cloves garlic, minced
• 1 tsp dried thyme
• Salt and pepper to taste
• Lemon wedges for serving

Instructions:

1. Preheat the oven to 400°F. Line a large baking sheet with parchment paper.

2. In a large bowl, toss the mixed vegetables and red onion with 1 tbsp of the olive oil, garlic, thyme, salt, and pepper.

3. Spread the seasoned vegetables in a single layer on the prepared baking sheet. Roast for 20•25 minutes, stirring halfway, until the vegetables are tender and lightly browned.

4. While the vegetables are roasting, place the cod fillets on a separate baking sheet. Brush the cod with the remaining 1 tbsp of olive oil and season with salt and pepper.

5. When the vegetables have about 10 minutes left to roast, add the cod to the oven and bake for 12•15 minutes, or until the cod is opaque and flakes easily with a fork.

6. Serve the baked cod immediately, topped with the roasted vegetables. Garnish with lemon wedges.

This baked cod with roasted vegetables dish is an excellent choice for the Galveston Diet during menopause. Cod is a lean, high•protein fish that is rich in omega•3 fatty acids, which can help support heart and brain health. The roasted vegetables provide a variety of vitamins, minerals, and antioxidants to support overall health.

The combination of the protein•rich cod and the fiber•rich vegetables makes this a filling and satisfying meal. Adjust the portion sizes as needed to fit your individual dietary needs during menopause.

16. Greek Salad with Grilled Chicken

Ingredients:

- 4 boneless, skinless chicken breasts
- 1 tbsp olive oil
- 1 tsp dried oregano
- Salt and pepper to taste
- 6 cups chopped romaine lettuce
- 1 cup cherry tomatoes, halved
- 1/2 cup diced cucumber
- 1/4 cup sliced red onion
- 1/4 cup pitted kalamata olives, halved
- 1/4 cup crumbled feta cheese
- 2 tbsp red wine vinegar
- 1 tbsp lemon juice
- 1 tbsp olive oil
- 1 tsp Dijon mustard
- 1 tsp dried oregano
- Salt and pepper to taste

Instructions:

1. Preheat grill or grill pan to medium·high heat.

2. Brush the chicken breasts with 1 tbsp of olive oil and season with 1 tsp dried oregano, salt, and pepper.

3. Grill the chicken for 5·7 minutes per side, or until cooked through. Let the chicken rest for 5 minutes, then slice or chop it.

4. In a large salad bowl, combine the chopped romaine lettuce, cherry tomatoes, cucumber, red onion, kalamata olives, and feta cheese.

5. In a small bowl, whisk together the red wine vinegar, lemon juice, 1 tbsp olive oil, Dijon mustard, 1 tsp dried oregano, salt, and pepper.

6. Drizzle the dressing over the salad and toss to coat. Top the salad with the grilled chicken slices. Serve the Greek salad with grilled chicken immediately.

This Greek salad with grilled chicken is a great option for the Galveston Diet during menopause. The lean protein from the chicken, healthy fats from the olive oil and olives, and fiber·rich vegetables make it a well·balanced and satisfying meal. The Mediterranean·inspired flavors also provide a variety of antioxidants and nutrients to support overall health during this stage of life.

17. Black Bean and Sweet Potato Tacos

Ingredients:

- 2 medium sweet potatoes, peeled and diced
- 1 tbsp olive oil
- 1 tsp chili powder
- 1/2 tsp cumin
- Salt and pepper to taste
- 1 (15 oz) can black beans, rinsed and drained
- 8•10 small corn tortillas
- 1 avocado, sliced
- 1/4 cup crumbled feta cheese
- 2 tbsp chopped fresh cilantro
- Lime wedges for serving

Instructions:

1. Preheat oven to 400°F. Line a baking sheet with parchment paper.

2. In a large bowl, toss the diced sweet potatoes with the olive oil, chili powder, cumin, salt, and pepper. Spread the seasoned sweet potatoes in a single layer on the prepared baking sheet.

3. Roast the sweet potatoes for 20•25 minutes, stirring halfway, until they are tender and lightly browned.

4. In a medium bowl, mash the black beans with a fork or potato masher.

5. To assemble the tacos, spread a spoonful of mashed black beans onto each corn tortilla. Top with the roasted sweet potatoes, sliced avocado, crumbled feta cheese, and chopped cilantro.

6. Serve the black bean and sweet potato tacos with lime wedges.

These black bean and sweet potato tacos are a great option for the Galveston Diet during menopause. The sweet potatoes provide complex carbohydrates, fiber, and important vitamins and minerals. The black beans are a good source of plant•based protein and fiber, which can help support digestive and heart health.

The healthy fats from the avocado and the tangy feta cheese add flavor and nutrition to this dish. You can adjust the portion sizes and toppings to your liking to make this a satisfying and balanced meal.

18. Tomato Basil Soup

Ingredients:

• 2 tbsp olive oil
• 1 onion, diced
• 3 cloves garlic, minced
• 2 (28 oz) cans diced tomatoes
• 2 cups low•sodium vegetable or chicken broth
• 1/4 cup fresh basil leaves, chopped
• 1 tsp dried oregano
• 1/4 tsp red pepper flakes (optional)
• Salt and pepper to taste
• 2 tbsp heavy cream or unsweetened almond milk (optional)

Instructions:

1. In a large pot or Dutch oven, heat the olive oil over medium heat. Add the diced onion and sauté for 5•7 minutes, until translucent.

2. Add the minced garlic and cook for 1 minute, until fragrant.

3. Pour in the canned diced tomatoes and their juices, along with the vegetable or chicken broth. Bring the mixture to a simmer.

4. Stir in the chopped fresh basil, dried oregano, and red pepper flakes (if using). Season with salt and pepper to taste.

5. Reduce the heat to low and let the soup simmer for 15•20 minutes, allowing the flavors to meld.

6. If desired, use an immersion blender or carefully transfer the soup to a blender and blend until smooth and creamy. Alternatively, leave the soup chunky.

7. Stir in the heavy cream or unsweetened almond milk (if using) just before serving. Serve the tomato basil soup warm, garnished with additional fresh basil leaves if desired.

This tomato basil soup is a great option for the Galveston Diet during menopause. The tomatoes provide a good source of lycopene, an antioxidant that may help reduce the risk of certain health conditions. The fresh basil and herbs add flavor and additional nutrients.

The soup can be enjoyed on its own or paired with a small salad or a slice of whole grain toast for a complete and satisfying meal. Adjust the portion sizes and toppings as needed to fit your individual dietary needs during menopause.

19. Turkey and Veggie Skewers

Ingredients:

- 1 lb ground turkey
- 1 zucchini, cut into 1·inch pieces
- 1 red bell pepper, cut into 1·inch pieces
- 1 red onion, cut into 1·inch pieces
- 8 cherry tomatoes
- 2 tbsp olive oil
- 1 tsp dried oregano
- 1 tsp garlic powder
- Salt and pepper to taste
- Wooden or metal skewers

Instructions:

1. Preheat your grill or grill pan to medium·high heat.

2. In a large bowl, mix the ground turkey with 1 tbsp of the olive oil, oregano, garlic powder, salt, and pepper until well combined.

3. Thread the turkey mixture, zucchini, bell pepper, onion, and cherry tomatoes onto the skewers, alternating the ingredients.

4. Brush the skewers with the remaining 1 tbsp of olive oil.

5. Grill the skewers for 12·15 minutes, turning occasionally, until the turkey is cooked through and the vegetables are tender.

6. Serve the turkey and veggie skewers immediately.

These turkey and veggie skewers are a great option for the Galveston Diet during menopause. The lean turkey provides a good source of protein, while the variety of vegetables offer fiber, vitamins, and antioxidants.

The combination of the protein and fiber·rich ingredients can help keep you feeling full and satisfied. You can adjust the types of vegetables used based on your preferences or what's in season.

Serve the skewers as a main dish or alongside a salad or roasted vegetables for a complete and balanced meal. The portion sizes can be adjusted to fit your individual dietary needs during menopause.

20. Roasted Brussels Sprouts with Balsamic Glaze

Ingredients:

- 1 lb Brussels sprouts, trimmed and halved
- 2 tbsp olive oil
- Salt and pepper to taste
- 2 tbsp balsamic vinegar
- 1 tbsp honey

Instructions:

1. Preheat your oven to 400°F. Line a baking sheet with parchment paper.

2. In a large bowl, toss the trimmed and halved Brussels sprouts with the olive oil, salt, and pepper until well coated.

3. Spread the Brussels sprouts in a single layer on the prepared baking sheet.

4. Roast the Brussels sprouts for 20•25 minutes, tossing halfway, until they are tender and lightly browned.

5. In a small saucepan, combine the balsamic vinegar and honey. Bring the mixture to a simmer over medium heat, stirring occasionally, until it thickens slightly, about 2•3 minutes.

6. Remove the roasted Brussels sprouts from the oven and drizzle the balsamic glaze over the top, tossing gently to coat.

7. Serve the roasted Brussels sprouts with balsamic glaze immediately.

This roasted Brussels sprouts dish is an excellent option for the Galveston Diet during menopause. Brussels sprouts are a nutrient•dense cruciferous vegetable that are high in fiber, vitamins, and antioxidants. The balsamic glaze adds a sweet and tangy flavor that complements the roasted Brussels sprouts perfectly.

The healthy fats from the olive oil, along with the fiber and nutrients from the Brussels sprouts, make this a filling and satisfying side dish or vegetarian main course. Adjust the portion sizes as needed to fit your individual dietary needs during menopause.

21. Spinach and Feta Stuffed Chicken Breast

Ingredients:

- 4 boneless, skinless chicken breasts
- 2 cups fresh spinach, chopped
- 1/2 cup crumbled feta cheese
- 2 tbsp olive oil
- 1 tsp dried oregano
- Salt and pepper to taste

Instructions:

1. Preheat your oven to 400°F. Lightly grease a baking dish or line a baking sheet with parchment paper.

2. Slice each chicken breast horizontally to create a pocket, being careful not to cut all the way through.

3. In a small bowl, mix together the chopped spinach and crumbled feta cheese.

4. Stuff the spinach and feta mixture evenly into the pockets of the chicken breasts.

5. Drizzle the stuffed chicken breasts with the olive oil and sprinkle with the dried oregano, salt, and pepper.

6. Bake the stuffed chicken breasts for 25•30 minutes, or until the chicken is cooked through and the internal temperature reaches 165°F.

7. Let the chicken rest for 5 minutes before serving.

This spinach and feta stuffed chicken breast is a great option for the Galveston Diet during menopause. The lean protein from the chicken, combined with the healthy fats from the olive oil and the fiber and nutrients from the spinach and feta, make this a well•balanced and satisfying meal.

The stuffing adds flavor and moisture to the chicken, and the dish can be easily customized by adjusting the amount of spinach and feta to your liking. Serve the stuffed chicken breasts with a side of roasted vegetables or a fresh salad for a complete and nutritious meal.

22. Chickpea Salad

Ingredients:

- 1 (15 oz) can chickpeas, rinsed and drained
- 1/2 cup diced cucumber
- 1/2 cup diced tomatoes
- 1/4 cup diced red onion
- 2 tbsp chopped fresh parsley
- 2 tbsp olive oil
- 1 tbsp lemon juice
- 1 tsp Dijon mustard
- 1/4 tsp ground cumin
- Salt and pepper to taste

Instructions:

1. In a large bowl, combine the rinsed and drained chickpeas, diced cucumber, tomatoes, red onion, and chopped parsley.

2. In a small bowl, whisk together the olive oil, lemon juice, Dijon mustard, and ground cumin. Season with salt and pepper to taste.

3. Pour the dressing over the chickpea salad and toss gently to coat everything evenly.

4. Refrigerate the chickpea salad for at least 30 minutes to allow the flavors to meld.

5. Serve the chickpea salad chilled or at room temperature.

This chickpea salad is a great option for the Galveston Diet during menopause. Chickpeas are a good source of plant·based protein, fiber, and complex carbohydrates, which can help support overall health and energy levels.

The fresh vegetables and herbs provide a variety of vitamins, minerals, and antioxidants, while the olive oil and lemon juice add healthy fats and a tangy flavor.

This salad can be enjoyed on its own as a light lunch or as a side dish. You can also add grilled chicken or tuna to make it a more substantial meal. Adjust the portion sizes as needed to fit your individual dietary needs during menopause.

23. Grilled Shrimp Skewers

Ingredients:

- 1 lb large shrimp, peeled and deveined
- 2 tbsp olive oil
- 2 tbsp lemon juice
- 1 tsp dried oregano
- 1/2 tsp garlic powder
- Salt and pepper to taste
- Wooden or metal skewers

Instructions:

1. If using wooden skewers, soak them in water for 30 minutes to prevent them from burning on the grill.

2. In a large bowl, combine the shrimp, olive oil, lemon juice, dried oregano, garlic powder, salt, and pepper. Toss to coat the shrimp evenly.

3. Thread the marinated shrimp onto the skewers, leaving a small space between each shrimp.

4. Preheat your grill or grill pan to medium•high heat.

5. Grill the shrimp skewers for 2•3 minutes per side, or until the shrimp are opaque and cooked through.

6. Serve the grilled shrimp skewers immediately, garnished with additional lemon wedges if desired.

These grilled shrimp skewers are a great option for the Galveston Diet during menopause. Shrimp is a lean protein source that is low in calories and high in nutrients, such as selenium and vitamin B12.

The marinade of olive oil, lemon juice, and herbs adds flavor and healthy fats to the dish. Grilling the shrimp keeps the cooking method simple and preserves the natural flavors.

You can serve the shrimp skewers as a main dish, accompanied by a side salad or roasted vegetables, or as a protein•rich appetizer. Adjust the portion sizes as needed to fit your individual dietary needs during menopause.

24. Caprese Salad with Balsamic Glaze

Ingredients:

• 8 oz fresh mozzarella cheese, sliced
• 2 large tomatoes, sliced
• 1/4 cup fresh basil leaves
• 2 tbsp olive oil
• 2 tbsp balsamic vinegar
• 1 tbsp honey
• Salt and pepper to taste

Instructions:

1. Arrange the sliced mozzarella and tomatoes on a serving platter or plate, alternating the layers.

2. Scatter the fresh basil leaves over the top of the salad.

3. In a small saucepan, combine the balsamic vinegar and honey. Bring the mixture to a simmer over medium heat, stirring occasionally, until it thickens slightly, about 2-3 minutes. Remove from heat and let cool slightly.

4. Drizzle the balsamic glaze over the Caprese salad.

5. Drizzle the olive oil over the salad and season with salt and pepper to taste.

6. Serve the Caprese salad with balsamic glaze immediately.

This Caprese salad is a great option for the Galveston Diet during menopause. The fresh mozzarella, tomatoes, and basil provide a variety of nutrients, including vitamins, minerals, and antioxidants.

The balsamic glaze adds a sweet and tangy flavor to the salad, while the olive oil provides healthy fats. This dish is light, refreshing, and can be enjoyed as a side or a main course.

The portion sizes can be adjusted to fit your individual dietary needs during menopause. You can also add grilled chicken or shrimp to make it a more substantial meal.

25. Ratatouille

Ingredients:

- 1 medium eggplant, diced
- 1 medium zucchini, diced
- 1 medium yellow squash, diced
- 1 red bell pepper, diced
- 1 onion, diced
- 3 cloves garlic, minced
- 2 tbsp olive oil
- 1 (14 oz) can diced tomatoes
- 2 tbsp chopped fresh basil
- 1 tsp dried oregano
- Salt and pepper to taste

Instructions:

1. In a large skillet or Dutch oven, heat the olive oil over medium heat.

2. Add the diced eggplant, zucchini, yellow squash, bell pepper, and onion. Sauté for 8•10 minutes, stirring occasionally, until the vegetables are tender.

3. Add the minced garlic and sauté for an additional 1•2 minutes, until fragrant.

4. Pour in the canned diced tomatoes, including the juices. Stir in the chopped fresh basil and dried oregano.

5. Season the ratatouille with salt and pepper to taste.

6. Reduce the heat to low and let the ratatouille simmer for 15•20 minutes, stirring occasionally, until the flavors have melded and the vegetables are very tender.

7. Serve the ratatouille warm, either as a main dish or as a side accompaniment.

This ratatouille dish is an excellent option for the Galveston Diet during menopause. It is packed with a variety of nutrient•dense vegetables, including eggplant, zucchini, squash, and bell peppers, which provide fiber, vitamins, and antioxidants.

The tomatoes and herbs add flavor and additional health benefits. Ratatouille can be enjoyed as a vegetarian main course or as a side dish to complement grilled or roasted proteins.

Adjust the portion sizes as needed to fit your individual dietary requirements during menopause. This dish can also be made ahead of time and reheated for a quick and easy meal.

26. Cucumber Avocado Salad

Ingredients:

- 2 medium cucumbers, diced
- 2 ripe avocados, diced
- 1/4 cup diced red onion
- 2 tbsp chopped fresh cilantro
- 2 tbsp olive oil
- 1 tbsp lime juice
- 1 tsp Dijon mustard
- Salt and pepper to taste

Instructions:

1. In a large bowl, combine the diced cucumbers, avocados, red onion, and chopped cilantro.

2. In a small bowl, whisk together the olive oil, lime juice, and Dijon mustard. Season with salt and pepper to taste.

3. Pour the dressing over the cucumber and avocado mixture and gently toss to coat everything evenly.

4. Refrigerate the salad for at least 30 minutes to allow the flavors to meld.

5. Serve the cucumber avocado salad chilled or at room temperature.

This cucumber avocado salad is a great option for the Galveston Diet during menopause. Cucumbers are low in calories and high in water content, providing hydration and fiber. Avocados are a rich source of healthy monounsaturated fats, which can help support heart health.

The combination of the crunchy cucumbers, creamy avocados, and tangy dressing makes this a refreshing and satisfying salad. The red onion and cilantro add additional flavor and nutrients.

This salad can be enjoyed as a light main dish or a side accompaniment to grilled or roasted proteins. Adjust the portion sizes as needed to fit your individual dietary requirements during menopause.

27. Baked Halibut with Herbs

Ingredients:

- 4 (6 oz) halibut fillets
- 2 tbsp olive oil
- 2 tbsp chopped fresh parsley
- 1 tbsp chopped fresh dill
- 1 tbsp chopped fresh thyme
- 1 tsp lemon zest
- Salt and pepper to taste
- Lemon wedges for serving

Instructions:

1. Preheat your oven to 400°F. Lightly grease a baking dish or line a baking sheet with parchment paper.

2. Place the halibut fillets in the prepared baking dish or on the baking sheet.

3. In a small bowl, mix together the olive oil, chopped parsley, dill, thyme, and lemon zest. Season with salt and pepper.

4. Spoon the herb mixture evenly over the top of the halibut fillets, gently pressing it into the fish.

5. Bake the halibut for 12•15 minutes, or until it flakes easily with a fork and is opaque throughout.

6. Serve the baked halibut with herbs immediately, garnished with lemon wedges.

This baked halibut with herbs is an excellent option for the Galveston Diet during menopause. Halibut is a lean, high•protein fish that is also a good source of omega•3 fatty acids, which can help support heart and brain health.

The fresh herbs and lemon zest add flavor and antioxidants to the dish, while the olive oil provides healthy fats. The simple preparation allows the natural flavors of the halibut to shine.

Serve the baked halibut with a side of roasted vegetables or a fresh salad for a complete and balanced meal. Adjust the portion sizes as needed to fit your individual dietary requirements during menopause.

28. Veggie and Hummus Wrap

Ingredients:

• 4 whole wheat tortillas or wraps
• 1 cup hummus (any flavor)
• 1 cup shredded carrots
• 1 cup thinly sliced cucumber
• 1 cup baby spinach or arugula
• 1/2 cup diced red bell pepper
• 2 tbsp crumbled feta cheese (optional)

Instructions:

1. Spread about 1/4 cup of hummus evenly onto each whole wheat tortilla or wrap.

2. Layer the shredded carrots, sliced cucumber, baby spinach or arugula, and diced red bell pepper on top of the hummus.

3. If using, sprinkle the crumbled feta cheese over the vegetables.

4. Fold the bottom of the tortilla or wrap up, then fold in the sides and continue rolling tightly to create a wrap.

5. Cut the wrap in half diagonally, if desired, and serve immediately.

This veggie and hummus wrap is a great option for the Galveston Diet during menopause. The whole wheat tortilla or wrap provides complex carbohydrates and fiber, while the hummus adds protein and healthy fats.

The variety of fresh vegetables, such as carrots, cucumber, spinach, and bell pepper, provide a range of vitamins, minerals, and antioxidants to support overall health. The optional feta cheese adds a tangy flavor and extra calcium.

This wrap can be enjoyed as a light lunch or a satisfying snack. You can adjust the fillings based on your preferences or what's in season. Serve the wrap with a side of fresh fruit or a small salad for a complete and balanced meal.

29. Stuffed Bell Peppers

Ingredients:

- 4 large bell peppers (any color)
- 1 lb ground turkey or lean ground beef
- 1 cup cooked quinoa
- 1 (15 oz) can diced tomatoes
- 1/2 cup diced onion

- 2 cloves garlic, minced
- 1 tsp dried oregano
- 1/2 tsp ground cumin
- Salt and pepper to taste
- 1/2 cup shredded mozzarella cheese (optional)

Instructions:

1. Preheat your oven to 375°F. Lightly grease a baking dish.

2. Cut the tops off the bell peppers and remove the seeds and membranes. Place the hollowed-out peppers in the prepared baking dish.

3. In a large skillet, cook the ground turkey or beef over medium heat until browned and crumbled, about 5-7 minutes. Drain any excess fat.

4. Add the diced onion and minced garlic to the skillet. Sauté for 2-3 minutes until the onion is translucent.

5. Stir in the cooked quinoa, diced tomatoes, dried oregano, cumin, salt, and pepper. Mix well and cook for an additional 2-3 minutes.

6. Spoon the turkey/quinoa mixture evenly into the hollowed-out bell peppers.

7. If using, sprinkle the shredded mozzarella cheese over the tops of the stuffed peppers.

8. Bake the stuffed peppers for 25-30 minutes, or until the peppers are tender and the filling is hot and bubbly. Serve the stuffed bell peppers warm.

These stuffed bell peppers are a great option for the Galveston Diet during menopause. The bell peppers provide fiber, vitamins, and antioxidants, while the ground turkey or beef and quinoa offer protein and complex carbohydrates to help keep you feeling full and satisfied.

The optional mozzarella cheese adds a creamy texture and extra calcium. Adjust the portion sizes and fillings as needed to fit your individual dietary requirements during menopause.

30. Greek Chicken Gyros

Ingredients:

- 1 lb boneless, skinless chicken breasts, cut into 1-inch pieces
- 2 tbsp olive oil
- 2 tbsp lemon juice
- 1 tsp dried oregano
- 1 tsp garlic powder
- Salt and pepper to taste
- 4 whole wheat pita breads
- 1 cup diced tomatoes
- 1 cup diced cucumber
- 1/4 cup crumbled feta cheese
- 1/4 cup thinly sliced red onion
- 1/2 cup plain Greek yogurt
- 1 tbsp chopped fresh dill

Instructions:

1. In a large bowl, combine the diced chicken, olive oil, lemon juice, dried oregano, garlic powder, salt, and pepper. Toss to coat the chicken evenly.

2. Heat a grill or grill pan over medium-high heat. Cook the marinated chicken for 5-7 minutes per side, or until cooked through.

3. Warm the whole wheat pita breads according to package instructions.

4. To assemble the gyros, place the grilled chicken in the center of each pita. Top with diced tomatoes, cucumber, crumbled feta cheese, and sliced red onion.

5. In a small bowl, mix together the plain Greek yogurt and chopped fresh dill. Drizzle the yogurt sauce over the gyros. Serve the Greek chicken gyros immediately.

These Greek chicken gyros are a great option for the Galveston Diet during menopause. The lean chicken provides a good source of protein, while the whole wheat pita, vegetables, and Greek yogurt sauce offer a balance of complex carbohydrates, fiber, and healthy fats.

The Mediterranean-inspired flavors from the lemon, oregano, and feta cheese make this a satisfying and flavorful meal. Adjust the portion sizes and toppings as needed to fit your individual dietary requirements during menopause.

31. Spinach and Mushroom Quiche

Ingredients:

- 1 pre•made whole wheat pie crust
- 1 tbsp olive oil
- 8 oz sliced mushrooms
- 3 cups fresh spinach, chopped
- 6 large eggs
- 1 cup unsweetened almond milk
- 1/2 cup shredded mozzarella cheese
- 1/4 cup grated Parmesan cheese
- 1 tsp dried thyme
- Salt and pepper to taste

Instructions:

1. Preheat your oven to 375°F.

2. In a skillet, heat the olive oil over medium heat. Add the sliced mushrooms and sauté for 5•7 minutes, until they are tender and lightly browned.

3. Add the chopped fresh spinach to the skillet and cook for 2•3 minutes, until the spinach is wilted. Remove from heat and let cool slightly.

4. In a large bowl, whisk together the eggs and almond milk. Stir in the sautéed mushrooms and spinach, shredded mozzarella, grated Parmesan, dried thyme, salt, and pepper.

5. Pour the egg mixture into the pre•made whole wheat pie crust.

6. Bake the quiche for 35•40 minutes, or until the center is set and the top is lightly golden. Allow the quiche to cool for 10 minutes before slicing and serving.

This spinach and mushroom quiche is a great option for the Galveston Diet during menopause. The whole wheat pie crust provides complex carbohydrates and fiber, while the eggs, cheese, and mushrooms offer protein and healthy fats.

The spinach adds important vitamins and minerals, making this a well•balanced and nutrient•dense dish. You can adjust the fillings based on your preferences or what's in season.

Serve the quiche with a side salad or roasted vegetables for a complete and satisfying meal. Adjust the portion sizes as needed to fit your individual dietary requirements during menopause.

32. Asparagus and Goat Cheese Frittata

Ingredients:

• 1 lb asparagus, trimmed and cut into 1•inch pieces
• 1 tbsp olive oil
• 8 large eggs
• 1/4 cup unsweetened almond milk
• 2 oz crumbled goat cheese
• 2 tbsp chopped fresh basil
• Salt and pepper to taste

Instructions:
1. Preheat your oven to 375°F.

2. In a 9•inch oven•safe skillet or pie dish, heat the olive oil over medium heat. Add the chopped asparagus and sauté for 5•7 minutes, until tender.

3. In a large bowl, whisk together the eggs and almond milk. Season with salt and pepper.

4. Pour the egg mixture over the sautéed asparagus in the skillet. Sprinkle the crumbled goat cheese and chopped fresh basil over the top.

5. Transfer the skillet to the preheated oven and bake for 18•22 minutes, or until the frittata is set and lightly golden on top.

6. Remove the frittata from the oven and let it cool for 5 minutes before slicing and serving.

This asparagus and goat cheese frittata is a great option for the Galveston Diet during menopause. Asparagus is a nutrient•dense vegetable that provides fiber, vitamins, and antioxidants.

The eggs offer a good source of protein, while the goat cheese adds a creamy texture and tangy flavor. The almond milk helps keep the frittata light and moist.

This dish can be enjoyed for breakfast, lunch, or dinner, and can be easily customized with different vegetables or herbs based on your preferences. Adjust the portion sizes as needed to fit your individual dietary requirements during menopause.

33. Blackened Tilapia with Mango Salsa

Ingredients:

For the Mango Salsa:
• 1 ripe mango, diced
• 1/2 cup diced red onion
• 1/4 cup chopped fresh cilantro
• 1 tbsp lime juice
• 1 tsp olive oil
• Salt and pepper to taste

For the Tilapia:
• 4 (6 oz) tilapia fillets
• 2 tsp blackened seasoning
(or a blend of chili powder,
cumin, garlic powder, and
paprika)
• 1 tbsp olive oil

Instructions:

1. Make the mango salsa: In a medium bowl, combine the diced mango, red onion, cilantro, lime juice, and olive oil. Season with salt and pepper to taste. Cover and refrigerate until ready to serve.

2. Preheat your oven to 400°F. Line a baking sheet with parchment paper.

3. Pat the tilapia fillets dry and season both sides generously with the blackened seasoning.

4. Heat the 1 tbsp of olive oil in a large skillet over medium•high heat. Add the seasoned tilapia fillets and cook for 2•3 minutes per side, until the fish is lightly blackened.

5. Transfer the seared tilapia to the prepared baking sheet. Bake for 8•10 minutes, or until the fish flakes easily with a fork. Serve the blackened tilapia immediately, topped with the fresh mango salsa.

This blackened tilapia with mango salsa is a great option for the Galveston Diet during menopause. Tilapia is a lean, mild•flavored fish that is high in protein and low in mercury.

The mango salsa provides a sweet and tangy contrast to the spicy blackened seasoning, while also adding vitamins, minerals, and antioxidants. The healthy fats from the olive oil and the fiber from the mango and onion make this a well•balanced and satisfying meal.

Serve the tilapia with a side of roasted vegetables or a fresh salad for a complete and nutritious dinner. Adjust the portion sizes as needed to fit your individual dietary requirements during menopause.

34. Mediterranean Chickpea Salad

Ingredients:

- 1 (15 oz) can chickpeas, rinsed and drained
- 1 cup diced cucumber
- 1/2 cup diced tomatoes
- 1/4 cup diced red onion
- 1/4 cup crumbled feta cheese
- 2 tbsp chopped fresh parsley
- 2 tbsp olive oil
- 1 tbsp lemon juice
- 1 tsp dried oregano
- Salt and pepper to taste

Instructions:

1. In a large bowl, combine the rinsed and drained chickpeas, diced cucumber, tomatoes, red onion, crumbled feta cheese, and chopped parsley.

2. In a small bowl, whisk together the olive oil, lemon juice, and dried oregano. Season with salt and pepper to taste.

3. Pour the dressing over the chickpea salad and toss gently to coat everything evenly.

4. Refrigerate the Mediterranean chickpea salad for at least 30 minutes to allow the flavors to meld.

5. Serve the salad chilled or at room temperature.

This Mediterranean chickpea salad is a great option for the Galveston Diet during menopause. Chickpeas are a good source of plant·based protein, fiber, and complex carbohydrates, which can help keep you feeling full and satisfied.

The fresh vegetables, tangy feta cheese, and Mediterranean·inspired dressing provide a variety of vitamins, minerals, and healthy fats to support overall health during this stage of life.

This salad can be enjoyed as a light main dish or a side accompaniment to grilled or roasted proteins. Adjust the portion sizes as needed to fit your individual dietary requirements during menopause.

35. Cauliflower Crust Pizza with Veggies

Ingredients:

For the Cauliflower Crust:
• 1 head of cauliflower, riced
(about 4 cups riced cauliflower)
• 1 egg, beaten
• 1/2 cup shredded mozzarella cheese
• 2 tbsp grated Parmesan cheese
• 1 tsp dried oregano
• 1/2 tsp garlic powder
• Salt and pepper to taste

For the Toppings:
• 1/2 cup marinara sauce
• 1 cup sliced mushrooms
• 1 cup diced bell peppers
• 1/2 cup sliced black olives
• 1 cup shredded mozzarella cheese

Instructions:

1. Preheat your oven to 400°F. Line a baking sheet with parchment paper.

2. To make the cauliflower crust, place the riced cauliflower in a microwave•safe bowl and microwave for 5•7 minutes, until tender. Allow to cool slightly.

3. Transfer the cooked cauliflower to a clean kitchen towel or cheesecloth and squeeze out as much moisture as possible.

4. In a bowl, mix the squeezed cauliflower, beaten egg, shredded mozzarella, Parmesan, oregano, garlic powder, salt, and pepper until well combined.

5. Press the cauliflower mixture onto the prepared baking sheet, forming a thin, even crust. Bake the cauliflower crust for 20•25 minutes, until golden brown and crispy.

7. Remove the crust from the oven and top with the marinara sauce, sliced mushrooms, bell peppers, black olives, and shredded mozzarella cheese.

8. Return the pizza to the oven and bake for an additional 10•15 minutes, or until the cheese is melted and bubbly. Slice and serve the cauliflower crust pizza immediately.

This cauliflower crust pizza is a great option for the Galveston Diet during menopause. The cauliflower crust provides a low•carb, gluten•free base, while the vegetable toppings offer a variety of nutrients and fiber.

The combination of the protein•rich cheese and the fiber•rich vegetables can help keep you feeling full and satisfied. Adjust the toppings based on your preferences or what's in season.

36. Broccoli and Cheddar Stuffed Chicken Breast

Ingredients:

- 4 boneless, skinless chicken breasts
- 1 cup chopped broccoli florets
- 1/2 cup shredded cheddar cheese
- 2 tbsp olive oil
- 1 tsp dried thyme
- Salt and pepper to taste

Instructions:

1. Preheat your oven to 400°F. Lightly grease a baking dish or line a baking sheet with parchment paper.

2. Slice each chicken breast horizontally to create a pocket, being careful not to cut all the way through.

3. In a small bowl, mix together the chopped broccoli florets and shredded cheddar cheese.

4. Stuff the broccoli and cheese mixture evenly into the pockets of the chicken breasts.

5. Drizzle the stuffed chicken breasts with the olive oil and sprinkle with the dried thyme, salt, and pepper.

6. Bake the stuffed chicken breasts for 25•30 minutes, or until the chicken is cooked through and the internal temperature reaches 165°F. Let the chicken rest for 5 minutes before serving.

This broccoli and cheddar stuffed chicken breast is a great option for the Galveston Diet during menopause. The lean protein from the chicken, combined with the fiber and nutrients from the broccoli, and the healthy fats from the olive oil, make this a well•balanced and satisfying meal.

The cheese adds creaminess and flavor to the dish, while the thyme provides an aromatic seasoning. This recipe can be easily customized by adjusting the amount of broccoli and cheese to your liking.

Serve the stuffed chicken breasts with a side of roasted vegetables or a fresh salad for a complete and nutritious dinner. Adjust the portion sizes as needed to fit your individual dietary requirements during menopause.

37. Spaghetti Squash with Marinara Sauce

Ingredients:

- 1 medium spaghetti squash, halved lengthwise and seeds removed
- 2 tbsp olive oil
- 1 onion, diced
- 3 cloves garlic, minced
- 1 (28 oz) can crushed tomatoes
- 1 tsp dried oregano
- 1/2 tsp dried basil
- Salt and pepper to taste
- Grated parmesan cheese for serving (optional)

Instructions:

1. Preheat oven to 400°F. Place the spaghetti squash halves cut•side down on a baking sheet. Bake for 40•50 minutes, until tender when pierced with a fork.

2. While the squash is baking, make the marinara sauce. In a large skillet, heat the olive oil over medium heat. Add the onion and sauté for 5 minutes until translucent.

3. Add the garlic and sauté for 1 minute until fragrant.

4. Pour in the crushed tomatoes and stir in the oregano, basil, salt and pepper. Simmer the sauce for 10•15 minutes, stirring occasionally, until thickened.

5. Once the squash is cooked, use a fork to scrape the flesh into spaghetti•like strands.

6. Serve the spaghetti squash strands topped with the warm marinara sauce. Sprinkle with parmesan cheese if desired.

Enjoy your healthy and delicious spaghetti squash meal!

38. Turkey Chili

Ingredients:

- 1 lb ground turkey
- 1 onion, diced
- 3 cloves garlic, minced
- 2 tbsp chili powder
- 1 tsp ground cumin
- 1 tsp dried oregano
- 1/2 tsp smoked paprika
- 1/4 tsp cayenne pepper (optional, for heat)
- 1 (15 oz) can diced tomatoes
- 1 (15 oz) can kidney beans, drained and rinsed
- 1 (15 oz) can black beans, drained and rinsed
- 1 cup low•sodium chicken or vegetable broth
- Salt and pepper to taste
- Toppings: shredded cheese, diced avocado, sour cream, chopped cilantro

Instructions:

1. In a large pot or Dutch oven, cook the ground turkey over medium•high heat, breaking it up with a wooden spoon, until browned, about 5•7 minutes. Drain any excess fat.

2. Add the onion and garlic to the pot and cook for 2•3 minutes until the onion is translucent.

3. Stir in the chili powder, cumin, oregano, smoked paprika, and cayenne (if using). Cook for 1 minute to toast the spices.

4. Pour in the diced tomatoes, kidney beans, black beans, and broth. Stir to combine.

5. Bring the chili to a simmer and let it cook for 20•25 minutes, stirring occasionally, until thickened.

6. Season with salt and pepper to taste.

7. Serve the turkey chili hot, topped with desired toppings like shredded cheese, diced avocado, sour cream, and chopped cilantro.

Enjoy this hearty and flavorful turkey chili! It's a great healthy weeknight meal.

39. Grilled Portobello Mushrooms with Balsamic Glaze

Ingredients:

- 4 large portobello mushroom caps, stems removed
- 2 tbsp olive oil
- 2 tbsp balsamic vinegar
- 1 tbsp honey
- 1 tsp dried thyme
- Salt and pepper to taste

Instructions:

1. Preheat grill or grill pan to medium·high heat.

2. In a small bowl, whisk together the olive oil, balsamic vinegar, honey, and thyme. Season with salt and pepper.

3. Brush the mushroom caps all over with the balsamic glaze mixture.

4. Grill the mushrooms for 4·5 minutes per side, basting with any remaining glaze, until tender and lightly charred.

5. Transfer the grilled mushrooms to a serving plate. Drizzle with any remaining balsamic glaze.

The Galveston Diet for menopause emphasizes anti·inflammatory foods like mushrooms, olive oil, and balsamic vinegar. This grilled portobello dish is a great option that aligns with the diet's guidelines:

- Portobello mushrooms are a good source of antioxidants, fiber, and B vitamins.
- Olive oil provides healthy monounsaturated fats.
- Balsamic vinegar is rich in polyphenols with anti·inflammatory properties.
- Honey adds a touch of sweetness without spiking blood sugar levels.

Serve these balsamic glazed grilled portobellos as a main dish or as a side to a lean protein. Enjoy this flavorful and nutritious menopausal·friendly recipe!

40. Tofu Stir•Fry with Broccoli

Ingredients:

• 1 block (14 oz) extra•firm tofu, pressed and cubed
• 2 tbsp sesame oil
• 3 cups broccoli florets
• 1 red bell pepper, sliced
• 3 cloves garlic, minced
• 1 tbsp grated fresh ginger
• 2 tbsp low•sodium soy sauce or tamari
• 1 tbsp rice vinegar
• 1 tsp honey
• Salt and pepper to taste
• Chopped green onions and sesame seeds for garnish (optional)

Instructions:

1. In a large skillet or wok, heat the sesame oil over medium•high heat.

2. Add the cubed tofu and stir•fry for 5•7 minutes, until lightly browned on all sides. Transfer the tofu to a plate.

3. Add the broccoli florets and bell pepper slices to the skillet. Stir•fry for 3•4 minutes until the vegetables are crisp•tender.

4. Add the garlic and ginger to the skillet and cook for 1 minute, until fragrant.

5. Return the tofu to the skillet. Pour in the soy sauce, rice vinegar, and honey. Toss everything together and cook for 2•3 minutes more, until heated through.

6. Season with salt and pepper to taste.

7. Serve the tofu stir•fry hot, garnished with chopped green onions and sesame seeds if desired.

This tofu and vegetable stir•fry aligns well with the Galveston Diet for menopause:

• Tofu is a great plant•based protein source.
• Broccoli and bell peppers are nutrient•dense vegetables.
• Sesame oil, soy sauce, and rice vinegar provide anti•inflammatory benefits.
• Honey adds a touch of sweetness without spiking blood sugar.

41. Cobb Salad with Grilled Chicken

Ingredients:

- 4 boneless, skinless chicken breasts
- 1 tbsp olive oil
- Salt and pepper to taste
- 8 cups chopped romaine lettuce
- 1 cup cherry tomatoes, halved
- 1 avocado, diced
- 2 hard·boiled eggs, chopped
- 4 slices cooked bacon, crumbled
- 1/2 cup crumbled blue cheese
- 2 tbsp chopped chives

Dressing:
- 2 tbsp red wine vinegar
- 1 tbsp Dijon mustard
- 1 tbsp olive oil
- 1 tbsp lemon juice
- 1 tsp honey
- Salt and pepper to taste

Instructions:

1. Preheat grill or grill pan to medium·high heat. Brush the chicken breasts with 1 tbsp olive oil and season with salt and pepper.

2. Grill the chicken for 5·7 minutes per side, until cooked through. Let rest for 5 minutes, then slice or chop the chicken.

3. In a large salad bowl, arrange the chopped romaine lettuce.

4. Top the lettuce with the grilled chicken, cherry tomatoes, avocado, hard·boiled eggs, crumbled bacon, blue cheese, and chives.

5. In a small bowl, whisk together the ingredients for the dressing. Drizzle the dressing over the salad just before serving and toss to coat.

This Cobb salad is a nutritious and satisfying meal, featuring:

- Grilled chicken for lean protein
- Romaine lettuce, tomatoes, and avocado for fiber and vitamins
- Hard·boiled eggs and bacon for healthy fats
- Blue cheese for calcium
- A light, tangy vinaigrette dressing

42. Veggie and Bean Burritos

Ingredients:

- 1 tbsp olive oil
- 1 onion, diced
- 1 red bell pepper, diced
- 2 cloves garlic, minced
- 1 (15 oz) can black beans, drained and rinsed
- 1 (15 oz) can pinto beans, drained and rinsed
- 1 tsp ground cumin
- 1 tsp chili powder
- 1/2 tsp dried oregano
- Salt and pepper to taste
- 6•8 whole wheat tortillas
- 1 cup shredded cheddar or Monterey Jack cheese
- Toppings: salsa, guacamole, sour cream, chopped cilantro

Instructions:

1. In a large skillet, heat the olive oil over medium heat. Add the diced onion and bell pepper. Sauté for 5•7 minutes until softened.

2. Add the minced garlic and sauté for 1 minute until fragrant.

3. Stir in the black beans, pinto beans, cumin, chili powder, oregano, salt, and pepper. Cook for 3•4 minutes, mashing some of the beans slightly, to heat through and combine the flavors.

4. Warm the tortillas according to package instructions.

5. Spoon the bean and veggie mixture onto the center of each tortilla. Top with shredded cheese.

6. Fold the bottom of the tortilla up, then fold in the sides and roll up tightly to create a burrito.

7. Serve the burritos warm, with desired toppings like salsa, guacamole, sour cream, and chopped cilantro.

These veggie and bean burritos are a delicious, nutritious, and satisfying meatless meal. The combination of beans, peppers, onions, and spices provides plenty of fiber, protein, and flavor. Customize the toppings to your liking!

43. Coconut Curry Shrimp

Ingredients:

- 1 lb large shrimp, peeled and deveined
- 1 tbsp coconut oil
- 1 onion, diced
- 3 cloves garlic, minced
- 1 tbsp grated fresh ginger
- 2 tsp yellow curry powder
- 1 tsp ground turmeric
- 1 (13.5 oz) can full•fat coconut milk
- 1 tbsp lime juice
- Salt and pepper to taste
- Chopped cilantro for garnish

Instructions:

1. In a large skillet or wok, heat the coconut oil over medium heat.

2. Add the diced onion and sauté for 3•4 minutes until translucent.

3. Stir in the minced garlic and grated ginger. Cook for 1 minute until fragrant.

4. Add the curry powder and turmeric. Stir to coat the onions and toast the spices for 1 minute.

5. Pour in the coconut milk and bring the mixture to a simmer.

6. Add the shrimp and cook for 5•7 minutes, stirring occasionally, until the shrimp are opaque and cooked through.

7. Remove from heat and stir in the lime juice. Season with salt and pepper to taste.

8. Serve the coconut curry shrimp warm, garnished with chopped cilantro.

This coconut curry shrimp dish aligns well with the Galveston Diet for menopause:

- Shrimp is a lean protein source.
- Coconut milk provides healthy fats.
- Turmeric and curry powder have anti•inflammatory properties.
- Ginger and lime add flavor without added sugars.

44. Greek Stuffed Peppers

Ingredients:

- 1 tsp dried basil
- 1/4 tsp crushed red pepper flakes (optional)
- 1 (14 oz) can diced tomatoes
- 1/2 cup crumbled feta cheese
- Salt and pepper to taste
- Chopped parsley for garnish

- 4 large bell peppers, halved lengthwise and seeds removed
- 1 lb ground turkey or ground chicken
- 1 cup cooked quinoa
- 1 onion, diced
- 3 cloves garlic, minced
- 1 tsp dried oregano

Instructions:

1. Preheat oven to 375°F. Place the bell pepper halves in a baking dish and set aside.

2. In a large skillet, cook the ground turkey or chicken over medium heat, breaking it up with a wooden spoon, until browned, about 5•7 minutes. Drain any excess fat.

3. Add the diced onion and minced garlic to the skillet. Sauté for 2•3 minutes until the onion is translucent.

4. Stir in the cooked quinoa, oregano, basil, and red pepper flakes (if using). Season with salt and pepper.

5. Spoon the turkey/chicken and quinoa mixture into the bell pepper halves, packing it in tightly.

6. Pour the diced tomatoes around the stuffed peppers in the baking dish. Cover the dish with foil and bake for 30•35 minutes, until the peppers are tender.

8. Remove the foil, sprinkle the feta cheese over the tops of the stuffed peppers, and bake for 5 more minutes. Garnish the stuffed peppers with chopped parsley before serving.

These Greek•inspired stuffed peppers are a great option for the Galveston Diet:

- Bell peppers are a nutrient•dense vegetable.
- Ground turkey or chicken provide lean protein.
- Quinoa is a whole grain with fiber and protein.
- Feta cheese adds calcium and healthy fats.
- Herbs and spices provide anti•inflammatory benefits.

45. Lemon Garlic Roasted Chicken

Ingredients:

- 1 (4•5 lb) whole chicken
- 3 tbsp olive oil
- 4 cloves garlic, minced
- 2 tbsp lemon juice
- 1 tsp lemon zest
- 1 tsp dried thyme
- 1 tsp dried rosemary
- Salt and pepper to taste
- Lemon wedges for serving

Instructions:

1. Preheat oven to 425°F. Pat the chicken dry with paper towels.

2. In a small bowl, mix together the olive oil, minced garlic, lemon juice, lemon zest, thyme, and rosemary. Season generously with salt and pepper.

3. Rub the lemon•garlic mixture all over the outside of the chicken, including under the skin if desired.

4. Place the chicken in a roasting pan or baking dish. Roast for 60•75 minutes, until the internal temperature reaches 165°F.

5. Let the chicken rest for 10 minutes before carving and serving.

6. Serve the lemon garlic roasted chicken warm, with lemon wedges on the side.

This lemon garlic roasted chicken aligns well with the Galveston Diet for menopause:

- Chicken is a lean protein source.
- Olive oil provides healthy monounsaturated fats.
- Lemon and garlic add flavor without added sugars.
- Herbs like thyme and rosemary have anti•inflammatory properties.

Pair the roasted chicken with roasted vegetables or a fresh salad for a complete, nutritious meal. The bright lemon and garlic flavors make this a delicious and diet•friendly option.

46. Shrimp and Avocado Salad

Ingredients:

- 1 lb cooked shrimp, peeled and deveined
- 2 avocados, diced
- 1 cup cherry tomatoes, halved
- 1/2 red onion, thinly sliced
- 1/4 cup chopped fresh cilantro
- 2 tbsp olive oil
- 2 tbsp lime juice
- 1 tsp Dijon mustard
- 1/2 tsp ground cumin
- Salt and pepper to taste

Instructions:

1. In a large bowl, gently toss together the cooked shrimp, diced avocado, cherry tomatoes, red onion, and chopped cilantro.

2. In a small bowl, whisk together the olive oil, lime juice, Dijon mustard, and cumin. Season the dressing with salt and pepper.

3. Pour the dressing over the shrimp and avocado salad and toss gently to coat.

4. Serve the shrimp and avocado salad chilled or at room temperature.

This shrimp and avocado salad is a great option for the Galveston Diet:

- Shrimp is a lean protein source.
- Avocado provides healthy monounsaturated fats.
- Cherry tomatoes and red onion add fiber and antioxidants.
- Cilantro, lime juice, and Dijon mustard provide anti•inflammatory benefits.
- The simple dressing is free of added sugars.

This salad can be enjoyed on its own or served over a bed of greens for a more substantial meal. It's a refreshing and nutritious option that aligns with the Galveston Diet guidelines.

Enjoy this flavorful and diet•friendly shrimp and avocado salad!

47. Quinoa Stuffed Bell Peppers

Ingredients:

• 4 large bell peppers, halved lengthwise and seeds removed
• 1 cup cooked quinoa
• 1 (15 oz) can black beans, drained and rinsed
• 1 cup diced tomatoes
• 1/2 cup crumbled feta cheese
• 1/4 cup chopped fresh parsley
• 2 cloves garlic, minced
• 1 tsp ground cumin
• 1/2 tsp dried oregano
• Salt and pepper to taste

Instructions:

1. Preheat oven to 375°F. Place the bell pepper halves in a baking dish and set aside.

2. In a large bowl, combine the cooked quinoa, black beans, diced tomatoes, feta cheese, parsley, minced garlic, cumin, and oregano. Season with salt and pepper.

3. Spoon the quinoa mixture evenly into the bell pepper halves, packing it in tightly.

4. Cover the baking dish with foil and bake for 30•35 minutes, until the peppers are tender.

5. Remove the foil and bake for an additional 5 minutes to lightly brown the tops. Serve the quinoa stuffed bell peppers warm.

This quinoa stuffed bell pepper dish aligns well with the Galveston Diet for menopause:

• Bell peppers are a nutrient•dense vegetable.
• Quinoa is a whole grain with fiber and protein.
• Black beans provide plant•based protein and fiber.
• Feta cheese adds calcium and healthy fats.
• Herbs and spices like parsley, garlic, cumin, and oregano have anti•inflammatory properties.

The combination of the bell peppers, quinoa, beans, and Mediterranean•inspired flavors makes this a delicious and nutritious meal option for the Galveston Diet. Enjoy these flavorful and diet•friendly stuffed peppers!

48. Veggie Stir•Fry with Tofu

Ingredients:

- 1 block (14 oz) extra•firm tofu, pressed and cubed
- 2 tbsp sesame oil
- 2 cups broccoli florets
- 1 red bell pepper, sliced
- 1 cup sliced mushrooms
- 1 cup snow peas or snap peas
- 3 cloves garlic, minced
- 1 tbsp grated fresh ginger
- 2 tbsp low•sodium soy sauce or tamari
- 1 tbsp rice vinegar
- 1 tsp sesame seeds (optional)
- Salt and pepper to taste

Instructions:

1. In a large skillet or wok, heat the sesame oil over medium•high heat.

2. Add the cubed tofu and stir•fry for 5•7 minutes, until lightly browned on all sides. Transfer the tofu to a plate.

3. Add the broccoli, bell pepper, mushrooms, and snow/snap peas to the skillet. Stir•fry for 4•5 minutes until the vegetables are crisp•tender.

4. Add the minced garlic and grated ginger to the skillet. Cook for 1 minute, until fragrant.

5. Return the tofu to the skillet. Pour in the soy sauce and rice vinegar. Toss everything together and cook for 2•3 minutes more, until heated through.

6. Remove from heat and sprinkle with sesame seeds, if using. Season with salt and pepper to taste. Serve the veggie and tofu stir•fry hot, over steamed brown rice or cauliflower rice if desired.

This veggie and tofu stir•fry aligns well with the Galveston Diet for menopause:

- Tofu is a plant•based protein source.
- Broccoli, bell pepper, mushrooms, and snow/snap peas provide fiber and antioxidants.
- Sesame oil, soy sauce, and rice vinegar offer anti•inflammatory benefits.
- Ginger adds flavor without added sugars.

49. Chicken and Vegetable Curry

Ingredients:

- 1 lb boneless, skinless chicken breasts, cubed
- 2 tbsp coconut oil
- 1 onion, diced
- 3 cloves garlic, minced
- 1 tbsp grated fresh ginger
- 2 tsp curry powder
- 1 tsp ground turmeric
- 1 tsp ground cumin
- 1 (13.5 oz) can full•fat coconut milk
- 1 cup diced tomatoes
- 2 cups mixed vegetables (such as cauliflower, broccoli, bell pepper, and spinach)
- 1 tbsp lime juice
- Salt and pepper to taste
- Chopped cilantro for garnish

Instructions:

1. In a large skillet or Dutch oven, heat the coconut oil over medium heat.

2. Add the cubed chicken and sauté for 5•7 minutes, until lightly browned on all sides. Transfer the chicken to a plate.

3. Add the diced onion to the skillet and sauté for 3•4 minutes until translucent.

4. Stir in the minced garlic and grated ginger. Cook for 1 minute until fragrant.

5. Add the curry powder, turmeric, and cumin. Stir to coat the onions and toast the spices for 1 minute.

6. Pour in the coconut milk and diced tomatoes. Bring the mixture to a simmer.

7. Add the mixed vegetables and the cooked chicken back to the skillet. Simmer for 10•15 minutes, until the vegetables are tender and the chicken is cooked through.

8. Remove from heat and stir in the lime juice. Season with salt and pepper to taste.

9. Serve the chicken and vegetable curry warm, garnished with chopped cilantro.

This curry dish aligns well with the Galveston Diet for menopause:

- Chicken is a lean protein source.
- Coconut milk provides healthy fats.
- Vegetables like cauliflower, broccoli, and bell pepper offer fiber and antioxidants.
- Spices like turmeric, cumin, and curry powder have anti•inflammatory properties.
- Lime juice adds flavor without added sugars.

50. Greek Lemon Chicken Soup (Avgolemono)

Ingredients:

• 6 cups low•sodium chicken broth
• 1 lb boneless, skinless chicken breasts, cubed
• 1 cup uncooked orzo pasta
• 2 eggs
• 1/4 cup fresh lemon juice
• 2 tbsp chopped fresh dill
• Salt and pepper to taste

Instructions:

1. In a large pot, bring the chicken broth to a boil over medium•high heat.

2. Add the cubed chicken and orzo pasta to the pot. Reduce heat to medium•low and simmer for 10•12 minutes, until the orzo is tender and the chicken is cooked through.

3. In a medium bowl, whisk together the eggs and lemon juice.

4. Slowly ladle about 1 cup of the hot broth from the pot into the egg•lemon mixture, whisking constantly. This will temper the eggs.

5. Slowly pour the egg•lemon mixture back into the pot, whisking constantly, to thicken the soup.

6. Remove the pot from heat and stir in the chopped fresh dill. Season with salt and pepper to taste. Serve the Greek lemon chicken soup warm.

This avgolemono soup aligns well with the Galveston Diet for menopause:

• Chicken is a lean protein source.
• Orzo pasta provides complex carbohydrates.
• Eggs add protein and healthy fats.
• Lemon juice provides vitamin C and anti•inflammatory benefits.
• Fresh dill is a source of antioxidants.

The combination of the chicken, broth, eggs, and lemon creates a creamy, tangy, and nourishing soup that is perfect for the Galveston Diet. Enjoy this comforting and diet•friendly Greek lemon chicken soup!

51. Cauliflower Alfredo Pasta

Ingredients:

- 1 head of cauliflower, cut into florets
- 1 cup unsweetened almond milk
- 2 cloves garlic, minced
- 2 tbsp olive oil
- 1/4 cup grated parmesan cheese
- 1 tsp dried thyme
- 1/2 tsp ground nutmeg
- Salt and pepper to taste
- 8 oz whole wheat pasta (such as linguine or fettuccine)
- Chopped parsley for garnish (optional)

Instructions:

1. Bring a large pot of salted water to a boil. Add the cauliflower florets and cook until very tender, about 10•12 minutes. Drain and set aside.

2. In a blender or food processor, combine the cooked cauliflower, almond milk, minced garlic, olive oil, parmesan cheese, thyme, and nutmeg. Blend until smooth and creamy. Season with salt and pepper to taste.

3. Bring the same pot of water back to a boil. Cook the whole wheat pasta according to package instructions until al dente. Drain the pasta and return it to the pot.

4. Pour the cauliflower Alfredo sauce over the cooked pasta and toss to coat evenly.

5. Serve the cauliflower Alfredo pasta warm, garnished with chopped parsley if desired.

This cauliflower Alfredo pasta dish aligns well with the Galveston Diet for menopause:

- Cauliflower is a nutrient•dense vegetable.
- Almond milk provides a dairy•free, low•fat alternative to traditional cream.
- Parmesan cheese adds calcium and healthy fats.
- Whole wheat pasta is a complex carbohydrate with fiber.
- Garlic, thyme, and nutmeg offer anti•inflammatory benefits.

The creamy cauliflower sauce provides a healthier take on traditional Alfredo, making this a delicious and diet•friendly pasta option. Enjoy this comforting and nutritious meal!

52. Stuffed Acorn Squash

Ingredients:

• 1 (15 oz) can black beans,
drained and rinsed
• 1 tsp ground cumin
• 1 tsp dried oregano
• 1/4 tsp cayenne pepper (optional)
• Salt and pepper to taste
• 1/2 cup crumbled feta cheese

• 2 acorn squash, halved lengthwise and
seeds removed
• 1 tbsp olive oil
• 1 lb ground turkey or ground chicken
• 1 onion, diced
• 2 cloves garlic, minced
• 1 cup cooked quinoa

Instructions:

1. Preheat oven to 400°F. Place the acorn squash halves cut•side down on a baking sheet. Bake for 30•40 minutes, until tender when pierced with a fork.

2. In a large skillet, heat the olive oil over medium heat. Add the ground turkey or chicken and cook, breaking it up with a wooden spoon, until browned, about 5•7 minutes.

3. Add the diced onion and minced garlic to the skillet. Sauté for 2•3 minutes until the onion is translucent.

4. Stir in the cooked quinoa, black beans, cumin, oregano, and cayenne (if using). Season with salt and pepper.

5. Flip the baked acorn squash halves over and scoop the turkey/chicken and quinoa mixture into the squash cavities, packing it in tightly.

6. Sprinkle the crumbled feta cheese over the tops of the stuffed squash.

7. Return the stuffed squash to the oven and bake for an additional 10•15 minutes, until the cheese is melted and lightly browned. Serve the stuffed acorn squash warm.

This stuffed acorn squash dish aligns well with the Galveston Diet for menopause:

• Acorn squash is a nutrient•dense winter squash.
• Ground turkey or chicken provide lean protein.
• Quinoa is a whole grain with fiber and protein.
• Black beans add plant•based protein and fiber.
• Feta cheese offers calcium and healthy fats.
• Spices like cumin and oregano have anti•inflammatory properties.

53. Grilled Swordfish with Mango Salsa

Ingredients:

For the Mango Salsa:
• 1 ripe mango, diced
• 1/2 red onion, finely chopped
• 1 jalapeño, seeded and finely chopped
• 1/4 cup chopped fresh cilantro
• 2 tbsp lime juice
• 1 tsp olive oil
• Salt and pepper to taste

For the Swordfish:
• 4 (6 oz) swordfish steaks
• 1 tbsp olive oil
• Salt and pepper to taste

Instructions:

1. Make the mango salsa: In a medium bowl, combine the diced mango, red onion, jalapeño, cilantro, lime juice, and olive oil. Season with salt and pepper to taste. Cover and refrigerate until ready to serve.

2. Preheat grill or grill pan to medium•high heat.

3. Pat the swordfish steaks dry and brush both sides with the 1 tbsp of olive oil. Season generously with salt and pepper.

4. Grill the swordfish for 4•5 minutes per side, until cooked through and opaque in the center.

5. Transfer the grilled swordfish to plates and top with the chilled mango salsa.

6. Serve the swordfish with the mango salsa immediately.

This grilled swordfish with mango salsa aligns well with the Galveston Diet for menopause:

• Swordfish is a lean, high•protein fish.
• Mango provides fiber, vitamins, and antioxidants.
• Red onion, jalapeño, and cilantro offer anti•inflammatory benefits.
• Lime juice adds flavor without added sugars.
• Olive oil is a healthy source of monounsaturated fats.

The bright, fresh flavors of the mango salsa complement the grilled swordfish perfectly. This is a delicious and nutritious meal option for the Galveston Diet.

54. Mediterranean Veggie Sandwich

Ingredients:

• 2 slices whole grain or sprouted bread
• 2 tbsp hummus
• 1/2 cup sliced cucumber
• 1/2 cup sliced tomatoes
• 1/4 cup crumbled feta cheese
• 1/4 cup sliced kalamata olives
• 2 tbsp chopped fresh basil or parsley
• 1 tsp olive oil
• 1 tsp balsamic vinegar
• Salt and pepper to taste

Instructions:
1. Toast the two slices of whole grain or sprouted bread.

2. Spread the hummus evenly over one slice of toast.

3. Layer the sliced cucumber, tomatoes, crumbled feta cheese, and kalamata olives on top of the hummus.

4. Drizzle the olive oil and balsamic vinegar over the vegetables.

5. Sprinkle the chopped fresh basil or parsley over the top. Season with salt and pepper to taste.

6. Top with the other slice of toast to create a sandwich. Cut the sandwich in half and serve immediately.

This Mediterranean veggie sandwich is a great option for the Galveston Diet:

• Whole grain or sprouted bread provides complex carbohydrates and fiber.
• Hummus is a source of plant•based protein and healthy fats.
• Cucumber, tomatoes, and olives offer antioxidants and anti•inflammatory benefits.
• Feta cheese adds calcium and healthy fats.
• Herbs like basil and parsley provide additional anti•inflammatory properties.
• Olive oil and balsamic vinegar make a simple, flavorful dressing.

This sandwich is a nutritious and satisfying meatless meal that aligns with the Galveston Diet guidelines. Enjoy this Mediterranean•inspired veggie sandwich!

55. Baked Eggplant with Tomato and Feta

Ingredients:

- 1 medium eggplant, sliced into 1/2•inch rounds
- 2 tbsp olive oil, plus more for drizzling
- 1 cup diced tomatoes
- 1/2 cup crumbled feta cheese
- 2 tbsp chopped fresh basil
- 1 clove garlic, minced
- Salt and pepper to taste

Instructions:

1. Preheat oven to 400°F. Line a baking sheet with parchment paper.

2. Arrange the eggplant slices in a single layer on the prepared baking sheet. Brush or drizzle the eggplant slices with 2 tbsp of olive oil, making sure to coat both sides.

3. Bake the eggplant for 20•25 minutes, flipping halfway, until tender and lightly browned.

4. In a small bowl, combine the diced tomatoes, crumbled feta cheese, chopped basil, and minced garlic. Season with salt and pepper.

5. Remove the baked eggplant slices from the oven and top each one with a spoonful of the tomato•feta mixture.

6. Drizzle a small amount of olive oil over the top of the eggplant and tomato•feta topping.

7. Return the baking sheet to the oven and bake for an additional 5•7 minutes, until the feta is lightly melted. Serve the baked eggplant with tomato and feta warm.

This baked eggplant dish aligns well with the Galveston Diet for menopause:

- Eggplant is a nutrient•dense vegetable.
- Tomatoes provide lycopene and other antioxidants.
- Feta cheese offers calcium and healthy fats.
- Fresh basil and garlic have anti•inflammatory properties.
- Olive oil is a source of monounsaturated fats.

The combination of the tender baked eggplant, juicy tomatoes, and creamy feta cheese creates a flavorful and nutritious meal that fits the Galveston Diet guidelines. Enjoy this Mediterranean•inspired baked eggplant dish!

56. Spicy Black Bean Soup

Ingredients:

- 2 tbsp olive oil
- 1 onion, diced
- 3 cloves garlic, minced
- 1 jalapeño, seeded and finely chopped
- 2 tsp ground cumin
- 1 tsp chili powder
- 1/2 tsp smoked paprika
- 2 (15 oz) cans black beans, drained and rinsed
- 4 cups low•sodium vegetable or chicken broth
- 1 (14.5 oz) can diced tomatoes
- 1 tsp lime juice
- Salt and pepper to taste
- Chopped cilantro for garnish (optional)

Instructions:

1. In a large pot or Dutch oven, heat the olive oil over medium heat. Add the diced onion and sauté for 3•4 minutes until translucent.

2. Stir in the minced garlic and chopped jalapeño. Cook for 1 minute until fragrant.

3. Add the cumin, chili powder, and smoked paprika. Stir to coat the onions and toast the spices for 1 minute.

4. Pour in the black beans, broth, and diced tomatoes. Bring the soup to a simmer.

5. Reduce heat to medium•low and let the soup simmer for 15•20 minutes, stirring occasionally, until slightly thickened.

6. Remove from heat and stir in the lime juice. Season with salt and pepper to taste. Ladle the spicy black bean soup into bowls and garnish with chopped cilantro, if desired.

This black bean soup aligns well with the Galveston Diet for menopause:

- Black beans are a great source of plant•based protein and fiber.
- Jalapeño, cumin, chili powder, and paprika provide anti•inflammatory benefits.
- Lime juice adds flavor without added sugars.
- The broth•based soup is low in calories and fat.

57. Turkey and Spinach Meatballs

Ingredients:

- 1 lb ground turkey
- 1 cup chopped fresh spinach
- 1/2 cup whole wheat breadcrumbs
- 1 egg, lightly beaten
- 2 cloves garlic, minced
- 2 tbsp grated Parmesan cheese
- 1 tsp dried oregano
- 1/2 tsp salt
- 1/4 tsp black pepper

Instructions:

1. Preheat oven to 400°F. Line a baking sheet with parchment paper.

2. In a large bowl, combine the ground turkey, chopped spinach, breadcrumbs, beaten egg, minced garlic, Parmesan cheese, oregano, salt, and pepper. Mix until well incorporated.

3. Scoop the turkey•spinach mixture by the tablespoonful and roll into small meatballs, about 1•inch in size.

4. Arrange the meatballs in a single layer on the prepared baking sheet.

5. Bake for 18•20 minutes, turning halfway, until the meatballs are cooked through and lightly browned. Serve the turkey and spinach meatballs warm, over zucchini noodles, spaghetti squash, or with a side salad.

These turkey and spinach meatballs align well with the Galveston Diet for menopause:

- Ground turkey is a lean protein source.
- Spinach is a nutrient•dense green that provides fiber, vitamins, and antioxidants.
- Whole wheat breadcrumbs offer complex carbohydrates.
- Parmesan cheese adds calcium and healthy fats.
- Herbs and spices like oregano, garlic, salt, and pepper have anti•inflammatory properties.

The combination of the turkey, spinach, and Mediterranean•inspired seasonings makes these meatballs a flavorful und nutritious option for the Galveston Diet. Enjoy these healthy and delicious turkey and spinach meatballs!

58. Roasted Butternut Squash Salad

Ingredients:

- 1/4 cup toasted pumpkin seeds
- 2 tbsp balsamic vinegar
- 1 tbsp Dijon mustard
- 1 tbsp honey
- 1 tbsp olive oil

- 1 medium butternut squash, peeled, seeded, and cubed
- 2 tbsp olive oil
- Salt and pepper to taste
- 5 oz mixed greens
- 1/2 cup crumbled feta cheese

Instructions:

1. Preheat oven to 400°F. Line a baking sheet with parchment paper.

2. Toss the cubed butternut squash with 2 tbsp of olive oil. Season with salt and pepper.

3. Roast the butternut squash for 25•30 minutes, stirring halfway, until tender and lightly browned.

4. Allow the roasted squash to cool slightly.

5. In a large salad bowl, combine the mixed greens, roasted butternut squash, crumbled feta cheese, and toasted pumpkin seeds.

6. In a small bowl, whisk together the balsamic vinegar, Dijon mustard, honey, and 1 tbsp olive oil. Season the dressing with salt and pepper.

7. Drizzle the balsamic dressing over the salad and toss gently to coat. Serve the roasted butternut squash salad immediately.

This butternut squash salad aligns well with the Galveston Diet for menopause:

- Butternut squash is a nutrient•dense winter squash.
- Mixed greens provide fiber and antioxidants.
- Feta cheese offers calcium and healthy fats.
- Pumpkin seeds are a source of anti•inflammatory omega•3s.
- The balsamic vinaigrette dressing is free of added sugars.

The combination of the roasted squash, greens, cheese, and seeds creates a flavorful and satisfying salad that fits the Galveston Diet guidelines. Enjoy this nutritious and delicious roasted butternut squash salad!

59. Lemon Herb Grilled Shrimp

Ingredients:

- 1 lb large shrimp, peeled and deveined
- 2 tbsp olive oil
- 2 tbsp lemon juice
- 2 tsp lemon zest
- 2 cloves garlic, minced
- 1 tbsp chopped fresh parsley
- 1 tbsp chopped fresh basil
- 1/2 tsp dried oregano
- Salt and pepper to taste
- Lemon wedges for serving

Instructions:

1. In a large bowl, combine the shrimp, olive oil, lemon juice, lemon zest, minced garlic, parsley, basil, and oregano. Toss to coat the shrimp evenly. Season with salt and pepper.

2. Preheat grill or grill pan to medium-high heat.

3. Thread the marinated shrimp onto metal or wooden skewers, leaving a little space between each shrimp.

4. Grill the shrimp skewers for 2-3 minutes per side, until the shrimp are opaque and cooked through.

5. Transfer the grilled lemon herb shrimp to a serving platter. Serve immediately with lemon wedges on the side.

This lemon herb grilled shrimp dish aligns well with the Galveston Diet for menopause:

- Shrimp is a lean protein source.
- Olive oil provides healthy monounsaturated fats.
- Lemon juice and zest add flavor without added sugars.
- Fresh herbs like parsley, basil, and oregano have anti-inflammatory properties.

The bright, Mediterranean-inspired flavors of the lemon, herbs, and garlic complement the grilled shrimp perfectly. This is a light, flavorful, and nutritious option that fits the Galveston Diet guidelines.

60. Portobello Mushroom Burger

Ingredients:

• 4 large portobello mushroom caps, stems removed
• 2 tbsp olive oil
• 1 tsp balsamic vinegar
• 1 tsp dried oregano
• Salt and pepper to taste
• 4 whole grain or sprouted buns
• 4 slices tomato
• 4 slices avocado
• 1/4 cup crumbled feta cheese

Instructions:

1. Preheat grill or grill pan to medium•high heat.

2. In a shallow dish, combine the olive oil, balsamic vinegar, and dried oregano. Season with salt and pepper.

3. Add the portobello mushroom caps to the dish and turn to coat both sides with the oil mixture.

4. Grill the marinated portobello caps for 4•5 minutes per side, until tender and lightly charred. Toast the whole grain or sprouted buns.

5. Place a grilled portobello mushroom cap on each bun bottom. Top with a slice of tomato, a slice of avocado, and a sprinkle of crumbled feta cheese. Add the bun tops and serve the portobello mushroom burgers immediately.

This portobello mushroom burger aligns well with the Galveston Diet for menopause:

• Portobello mushrooms are a nutrient•dense, meaty vegetable.
• Olive oil and balsamic vinegar provide healthy fats and anti•inflammatory benefits.
• Whole grain or sprouted buns are a complex carbohydrate source.
• Tomatoes, avocado, and feta cheese offer additional vitamins, minerals, and healthy fats.

The grilled, marinated portobello caps make a delicious and satisfying meatless burger option. Enjoy this flavorful and nutritious portobello mushroom burger as part of your Galveston Diet meal plan.

61. Thai Peanut Chicken Salad

Ingredients:

For the Peanut Dressing:
• 2 tbsp natural peanut butter
• 2 tbsp rice vinegar
• 1 tbsp low•sodium soy sauce
• 1 tbsp lime juice
• 1 tsp sesame oil
• 1 tsp honey
• 1 tsp grated fresh ginger
• 1 clove garlic, minced
• 2•3 tbsp water to thin

For the Salad:
• 4 cups shredded cooked chicken
• 4 cups mixed greens
• 1 cup shredded red cabbage
• 1 cup shredded carrots
• 1/2 cup chopped cucumber
• 2 tbsp chopped fresh cilantro
• 2 tbsp chopped roasted peanuts

Instructions:

1. In a large salad bowl, combine the shredded chicken, mixed greens, red cabbage, carrots, cucumber, cilantro, and chopped peanuts.

2. In a small bowl, whisk together all the ingredients for the peanut dressing, adding water as needed to thin it to a pourable consistency.

3. Drizzle the peanut dressing over the salad and toss gently to coat.

4. Serve the Thai peanut chicken salad immediately.

This Thai•inspired salad aligns well with the Galveston Diet for menopause:

• Chicken is a lean protein source.
• Mixed greens, cabbage, and carrots provide fiber and antioxidants.
• Peanut butter offers healthy fats and plant•based protein.
• Sesame oil, ginger, and garlic have anti•inflammatory properties.
• Lime juice and rice vinegar add flavor without added sugars.

The combination of the flavorful peanut dressing and the crunchy, nutrient•dense vegetables and chicken makes this a satisfying and diet•friendly salad option. Enjoy this Thai peanut chicken salad as part of your Galveston Diet meal plan.

62. Veggie and Quinoa Stuffed Mushrooms

Ingredients:

• 12 large cremini or button mushrooms, stems removed and finely chopped
• 1 tbsp olive oil
• 1/2 cup diced onion
• 2 cloves garlic, minced
• 1/2 cup cooked quinoa
• 1/2 cup diced bell pepper
• 2 tbsp chopped fresh parsley
• 1 tbsp grated Parmesan cheese
• Salt and pepper to taste

Instructions:

1. Preheat oven to 375°F. Lightly grease a baking sheet.

2. Arrange the mushroom caps, stem•side up, on the prepared baking sheet.

3. In a skillet, heat the olive oil over medium heat. Add the chopped mushroom stems, diced onion, and minced garlic. Sauté for 3•4 minutes until softened.

4. Stir in the cooked quinoa, diced bell pepper, and chopped parsley. Season with salt and pepper.

5. Spoon the quinoa and vegetable mixture evenly into the mushroom caps, packing it in gently. Sprinkle the grated Parmesan cheese over the tops of the stuffed mushrooms.

6. Bake for 15•18 minutes, until the mushrooms are tender and the filling is hot. Serve the veggie and quinoa stuffed mushrooms warm.

This stuffed mushroom dish aligns well with the Galveston Diet for menopause:

• Mushrooms are a nutrient•dense vegetable.
• Quinoa is a whole grain with fiber and protein.
• Bell peppers provide vitamins and antioxidants.
• Parsley and Parmesan cheese offer anti•inflammatory benefits.
• The dish is low in calories and fat.

The combination of the savory quinoa and vegetable filling with the tender baked mushrooms makes these stuffed mushrooms a delicious and nutritious option for the Galveston Diet. Enjoy this flavorful and diet•friendly appetizer or side dish!

63. Baked Chicken with Brussels Sprouts and Bacon

Ingredients:

- 4 boneless, skinless chicken breasts
- 1 lb brussels sprouts, trimmed and halved
- 4 slices bacon, chopped
- 2 tbsp olive oil
- 1 tsp garlic powder
- 1 tsp dried thyme
- Salt and pepper to taste

Instructions:

1. Preheat oven to 400°F. Line a large baking sheet with parchment paper.

2. In a large bowl, toss the brussels sprouts and chopped bacon with 1 tbsp of the olive oil. Season with salt and pepper. Spread out on one side of the prepared baking sheet.

3. In the same bowl, toss the chicken breasts with the remaining 1 tbsp olive oil, garlic powder, and dried thyme. Season with salt and pepper.

4. Place the chicken on the other side of the baking sheet, keeping it separate from the brussels sprouts.

5. Bake for 25•30 minutes, until the chicken is cooked through and the brussels sprouts are tender and lightly browned.

6. Serve the baked chicken immediately, with the roasted brussels sprouts and bacon on the side.

Enjoy your delicious and healthy baked chicken dinner!

64. Mediterranean Stuffed Zucchini

Ingredients:

• 4 medium zucchini, halved lengthwise
• 1 tbsp olive oil
• 1 onion, diced
• 3 cloves garlic, minced
• 1 lb ground lamb or ground beef
• 1 cup cooked quinoa
• 1 cup crumbled feta cheese
• 1/4 cup chopped fresh parsley
• 1 tsp dried oregano
• Salt and pepper to taste
• 1/4 cup grated Parmesan cheese

Instructions:

1. Preheat oven to 375°F. Scoop out the flesh from the zucchini halves, leaving about 1/4 inch of the shell. Finely chop the zucchini flesh.

2. In a skillet, heat the olive oil over medium heat. Add the onion and sauté for 3•4 minutes until translucent. Add the garlic and chopped zucchini flesh and cook for 2•3 more minutes.

3. Add the ground lamb/beef to the skillet and cook, breaking it up with a spoon, until browned and cooked through, about 5•7 minutes. Drain any excess fat.

4. Remove from heat and stir in the cooked quinoa, feta, parsley, oregano, salt and pepper.

5. Arrange the zucchini halves in a baking dish. Stuff each half evenly with the meat and quinoa mixture.

6. Top with the grated Parmesan cheese.

7. Bake for 25•30 minutes, until the zucchini is tender and the filling is hot.

8. Serve the Mediterranean stuffed zucchini warm, garnished with extra parsley if desired.

Enjoy this healthy and flavorful Mediterranean•inspired stuffed zucchini dish!

65. Salmon Cakes with Avocado Aioli

Ingredients:

For the Salmon Cakes:
- 1 (15 oz) can wild•caught salmon, drained and flaked
- 1 egg, lightly beaten
- 1/4 cup almond flour
- 2 tbsp chopped fresh parsley
- 1 tsp Dijon mustard
- 1/4 tsp salt
- 1/4 tsp black pepper
- 1 tbsp olive oil for cooking

For the Avocado Aioli:
- 1 ripe avocado, pitted and mashed
- 1/4 cup olive oil mayonnaise
- 1 tbsp lemon juice
- 1 garlic clove, minced
- 1/4 tsp salt
- 1/4 tsp black pepper

Instructions:

1. Make the salmon cakes: In a medium bowl, gently mix together the flaked salmon, egg, almond flour, parsley, Dijon, salt and pepper until well combined.

2. Form the mixture into 4•6 patties, about 1/2 inch thick.

3. In a skillet, heat the 1 tbsp olive oil over medium heat. Cook the salmon cakes for 3•4 minutes per side until golden brown.

4. Make the avocado aioli: In a small bowl, mash the avocado. Stir in the mayonnaise, lemon juice, garlic, salt and pepper until well combined.

5. Serve the warm salmon cakes topped with the avocado aioli. Enjoy!

This recipe is perfect for the Galveston Diet, as it features heart•healthy salmon, avocado, and olive oil • all great choices for women going through menopause. The salmon cakes provide lean protein, while the avocado aioli adds healthy fats.

66. Spinach and Artichoke Stuffed Chicken Breast

Ingredients:

• 4 boneless, skinless chicken breasts
• 1 (14 oz) can artichoke hearts, drained and chopped
• 1 cup fresh spinach, chopped
• 1/2 cup shredded mozzarella cheese
• 2 tbsp cream cheese, softened
• 2 tbsp grated Parmesan cheese
• 1 garlic clove, minced
• 1/4 tsp salt
• 1/4 tsp black pepper

Instructions:

1. Preheat oven to 375°F. Lightly grease a baking dish.

2. In a medium bowl, mix together the chopped artichoke hearts, spinach, mozzarella, cream cheese, Parmesan, garlic, salt and pepper until well combined.

3. Slice each chicken breast horizontally to create a pocket. Stuff each pocket evenly with the spinach and artichoke mixture.

4. Place the stuffed chicken breasts in the prepared baking dish.

5. Bake for 25•30 minutes, until the chicken is cooked through and the filling is hot.

6. Serve the spinach and artichoke stuffed chicken breasts warm.

This recipe is a great option for the Galveston Diet, as it features lean protein from the chicken, healthy fats from the olive oil and avocado, and nutrient•dense vegetables like spinach and artichoke hearts. The combination of flavors and textures makes it a delicious and satisfying meal for women going through menopause.

67. Eggplant Caponata

Ingredients:

- 1 medium eggplant, diced
- 2 tbsp olive oil
- 1 onion, diced
- 3 cloves garlic, minced
- 1 (14 oz) can diced tomatoes
- 2 tbsp red wine vinegar
- 2 tbsp capers, rinsed and drained
- 1/4 cup pitted and chopped green olives
- 2 tbsp chopped fresh basil
- 1 tsp dried oregano
- 1/4 tsp red pepper flakes (optional)
- Salt and pepper to taste

Instructions:

1. In a large skillet, heat the olive oil over medium heat. Add the diced eggplant and sauté for 5•7 minutes, until softened.

2. Add the onion and garlic to the skillet and cook for 2•3 minutes more, until the onion is translucent.

3. Stir in the diced tomatoes, red wine vinegar, capers, olives, basil, oregano, and red pepper flakes (if using). Season with salt and pepper.

4. Reduce heat to low and let the caponata simmer for 15•20 minutes, stirring occasionally, until the flavors have melded and the mixture has thickened.

5. Serve the eggplant caponata warm or at room temperature, as a side dish or appetizer. It can also be served over grilled fish or chicken.

This eggplant caponata recipe is perfect for the Galveston Diet, as it is packed with nutrient•dense vegetables, healthy fats from the olive oil, and anti•inflammatory herbs and spices. The combination of flavors makes it a delicious and satisfying option for women going through menopause.

68. Black Bean and Corn Salad

Ingredients:

- 1 (15 oz) can black beans, rinsed and drained
- 1 (15 oz) can corn, drained
- 1 red bell pepper, diced
- 1 cup cherry tomatoes, halved
- 1/2 red onion, diced
- 1/4 cup chopped fresh cilantro
- 2 tbsp olive oil
- 2 tbsp lime juice
- 1 tsp ground cumin
- 1/2 tsp chili powder
- Salt and pepper to taste

Instructions:

1. In a large bowl, combine the rinsed and drained black beans, drained corn, diced red bell pepper, halved cherry tomatoes, and diced red onion.

2. In a small bowl, whisk together the olive oil, lime juice, cumin, chili powder, salt, and pepper.

3. Pour the dressing over the black bean and corn mixture and toss gently to coat.

4. Stir in the chopped fresh cilantro.

5. Refrigerate the salad for at least 30 minutes to allow the flavors to meld.

6. Serve chilled or at room temperature.

This black bean and corn salad is a refreshing and flavorful side dish or light main course. It's packed with fiber, protein, and antioxidants from the vegetables and beans. The lime juice, cumin, and chili powder give it a nice Southwestern flair.

This salad is a great option for the Galveston Diet, as it is plant·based, low in calories, and full of nutrients that are beneficial for women during menopause.

69. Grilled Mahi Mahi with Pineapple Salsa

Ingredients:

For the Pineapple Salsa:
• 1 cup diced fresh pineapple
• 1/2 red onion, diced
• 1 jalapeño, seeded and minced
• 2 tbsp chopped fresh cilantro
• 1 tbsp lime juice
• 1/4 tsp salt

For the Mahi Mahi:
• 4 (6 oz) mahi mahi fillets
• 1 tbsp olive oil
• 1 tsp chili powder
• 1/2 tsp garlic powder
• 1/4 tsp salt
• 1/4 tsp black pepper

Instructions:

1. Make the pineapple salsa: In a medium bowl, combine the diced pineapple, red onion, jalapeño, cilantro, lime juice, and 1/4 tsp salt. Stir to mix well and set aside.

2. Prepare the mahi mahi: Pat the fillets dry and brush both sides with the olive oil. Season with the chili powder, garlic powder, salt, and pepper.

3. Preheat a grill or grill pan to medium•high heat. Grill the mahi mahi for 3•4 minutes per side, until cooked through and flaky.

4. Serve the grilled mahi mahi immediately, topped with the pineapple salsa.

This recipe is perfect for the Galveston Diet, as it features heart•healthy mahi mahi, fresh pineapple, and anti•inflammatory spices. The pineapple salsa adds a bright, tropical flavor that complements the grilled fish. This dish is low in calories and carbs, while providing lean protein, healthy fats, and essential nutrients that are beneficial for women during menopause.

70. Veggie and Lentil Soup

Ingredients:

• 1 tbsp olive oil
• 1 onion, diced
• 3 cloves garlic, minced
• 2 carrots, peeled and diced
• 2 celery stalks, diced
• 1 cup green beans, trimmed and cut into 1•inch pieces
• 1 cup diced zucchini
• 1 cup dried brown or green lentils, rinsed
• 6 cups low•sodium vegetable broth
• 1 (14 oz) can diced tomatoes
• 2 tsp dried thyme
• 1 tsp dried oregano
• Salt and pepper to taste
• Chopped fresh parsley for garnish (optional)

Instructions:

1. In a large pot or Dutch oven, heat the olive oil over medium heat. Add the onion and sauté for 3•4 minutes until translucent.

2. Add the garlic, carrots, celery, green beans, and zucchini. Sauté for 5•7 minutes, stirring occasionally, until the vegetables start to soften.

3. Stir in the lentils, vegetable broth, diced tomatoes, thyme, and oregano. Season with salt and pepper.

4. Bring the soup to a boil, then reduce heat and let it simmer for 25•30 minutes, until the lentils are tender.

5. Taste and adjust seasoning as needed.

6. Serve the veggie and lentil soup hot, garnished with chopped fresh parsley if desired.

This hearty, plant•based soup is an excellent choice for the Galveston Diet. It's packed with fiber, protein, and a variety of nutrient•dense vegetables. The lentils provide a good source of plant•based protein, while the olive oil and vegetables offer anti•inflammatory benefits. This soup is low in calories and carbs, making it a great option for women during menopause.

71. Turkey and Veggie Lettuce Wraps

Ingredients:

- 1 lb ground turkey
- 1 tbsp olive oil
- 1 onion, diced
- 2 cloves garlic, minced
- 1 cup diced mushrooms
- 1 cup diced bell pepper
- 1 cup shredded carrots
- 2 tbsp low•sodium soy sauce or tamari
- 1 tsp ground ginger
- 1/4 tsp red pepper flakes (optional)
- Salt and pepper to taste
- 12•16 large lettuce leaves (such as romaine or bibb)

For the Avocado Sauce:

- 1 ripe avocado, pitted and mashed
- 2 tbsp olive oil mayonnaise
- 1 tbsp lime juice
- 1 tbsp chopped fresh cilantro
- 1 garlic clove, minced
- Salt and pepper to taste

Instructions:

1. In a large skillet, cook the ground turkey over medium•high heat, breaking it up with a wooden spoon, until browned and cooked through, about 5•7 minutes. Drain any excess fat.

2. Add the olive oil to the skillet. Sauté the onion, garlic, mushrooms, bell pepper, and carrots for 5•7 minutes, until the vegetables are tender.

3. Stir in the soy sauce, ground ginger, and red pepper flakes (if using). Season with salt and pepper.

4. Make the avocado sauce: In a small bowl, mash the avocado. Stir in the mayonnaise, lime juice, cilantro, garlic, salt, and pepper.

5. To serve, place a spoonful of the turkey and veggie mixture into a lettuce leaf. Top with a dollop of the avocado sauce. Enjoy the turkey and veggie lettuce wraps immediately.

This recipe is perfect for the Galveston Diet, as it features lean protein from the turkey, healthy fats from the avocado and olive oil, and a variety of nutrient•dense vegetables. The lettuce wraps provide a low•carb, gluten•free option that is satisfying and delicious.

72. Quinoa and Roasted Vegetable Salad

Ingredients:

- 1 cup uncooked quinoa, rinsed
- 2 cups low•sodium vegetable broth
- 1 medium zucchini, diced
- 1 red bell pepper, diced
- 1 cup diced eggplant
- 1 red onion, diced
- 2 tbsp olive oil
- 1 tsp dried oregano
- 1/2 tsp garlic powder
- Salt and pepper to taste
- 2 tbsp balsamic vinegar
- 2 tbsp chopped fresh parsley
- 2 tbsp chopped fresh basil

Instructions:

1. Preheat oven to 400°F. Line a large baking sheet with parchment paper.

2. In a medium saucepan, combine the quinoa and vegetable broth. Bring to a boil, then reduce heat to low, cover and simmer for 15•20 minutes, until quinoa is cooked through. Fluff with a fork and set aside.

3. In a large bowl, toss the diced zucchini, bell pepper, eggplant, and onion with the olive oil, oregano, garlic powder, salt and pepper.

4. Spread the vegetables in a single layer on the prepared baking sheet. Roast for 20•25 minutes, stirring halfway, until tender and lightly browned.

5. In a large bowl, combine the cooked quinoa and roasted vegetables. Drizzle with the balsamic vinegar and toss to coat.

6. Stir in the chopped parsley and basil. Serve the quinoa and roasted vegetable salad warm or chilled.

This salad is an excellent choice for the Galveston Diet, as it is packed with fiber, protein, and antioxidants from the quinoa, vegetables, and herbs. The roasted vegetables add depth of flavor, while the balsamic vinegar provides a tangy note. This dish is low in calories and carbs, making it a nutritious and satisfying option for women during menopause.

73. Lemon Garlic Shrimp Pasta

Ingredients:

• 8 oz whole wheat pasta (such as linguine or spaghetti)
• 1 lb shrimp, peeled and deveined
• 2 tbsp olive oil
• 3 cloves garlic, minced
• 1/4 cup dry white wine or low•sodium chicken broth
• 2 tbsp lemon juice
• 1 tsp lemon zest
• 1/4 cup chopped fresh parsley
• Salt and pepper to taste

Instructions:

1. Bring a large pot of salted water to a boil. Cook the pasta according to package instructions until al dente. Drain and set aside.

2. In a large skillet, heat the olive oil over medium•high heat. Add the shrimp and garlic, and sauté for 2•3 minutes until the shrimp start to turn pink.

3. Pour in the white wine (or chicken broth) and lemon juice. Simmer for 2•3 minutes, until the shrimp are cooked through.

4. Remove the skillet from heat and stir in the cooked pasta, lemon zest, and chopped parsley. Toss to combine.

5. Season the lemon garlic shrimp pasta with salt and pepper to taste.

6. Serve the pasta warm, garnished with additional parsley if desired.

This recipe is a great option for the Galveston Diet, as it features lean protein from the shrimp, whole wheat pasta for fiber, and healthy fats from the olive oil. The lemon and garlic provide anti•inflammatory benefits, while the parsley adds antioxidants. This dish is low in calories and carbs, making it a nutritious and satisfying meal for women during menopause.

74. Greek Turkey Burgers with Tzatziki Sauce

Ingredients:

For the Turkey Burgers:
• 1 lb ground turkey
• 1/4 cup crumbled feta cheese
• 2 tbsp chopped fresh parsley
• 1 tsp dried oregano
• 1 garlic clove, minced
• 1/4 tsp salt
• 1/4 tsp black pepper

For the Tzatziki Sauce:
• 1 cup plain Greek yogurt
• 1/2 cucumber, peeled, seeded and grated
• 1 garlic clove, minced
• 1 tbsp lemon juice
• 1 tbsp chopped fresh dill
• 1/4 tsp salt

To Serve:
• 4 whole wheat pita rounds, halved
• Lettuce leaves
• Sliced tomatoes
• Sliced red onion

Instructions:

1. Make the turkey burgers: In a bowl, gently mix together the ground turkey, feta, parsley, oregano, garlic, salt, and pepper until just combined. Form into 4 equal•sized patties.

2. Make the tzatziki sauce: In a small bowl, stir together the Greek yogurt, grated cucumber, garlic, lemon juice, dill, and salt. Cover and refrigerate until ready to serve.

3. Preheat a grill or grill pan to medium•high heat. Cook the turkey burgers for 4•5 minutes per side, until cooked through.

4. To serve, place each turkey burger in a pita half. Top with lettuce, tomato, onion, and a generous dollop of the tzatziki sauce.

These Greek•inspired turkey burgers are a perfect choice for the Galveston Diet. The lean turkey provides protein, while the feta, yogurt, and vegetables offer important nutrients and anti•inflammatory benefits. The tzatziki sauce adds a refreshing, creamy topping. Serve with a side salad for a complete and satisfying meal.

75. Stuffed Cabbage Rolls

Ingredients:

- 1 medium head green cabbage
- 1 lb ground turkey
- 1 cup cooked brown rice
- 1 onion, finely chopped
- 2 cloves garlic, minced
- 1 tsp dried oregano
- 1/2 tsp dried thyme
- 1/4 tsp red pepper flakes (optional)
- Salt and pepper to taste
- 1 (15 oz) can tomato sauce
- 1 (14 oz) can diced tomatoes
- 2 tbsp lemon juice

Instructions:

1. Bring a large pot of water to a boil. Add the whole head of cabbage and cook for 5•7 minutes, until the outer leaves are softened. Remove the cabbage and let cool slightly.

2. Carefully peel off the softened cabbage leaves, keeping them intact. You should have about 12•14 leaves.

3. In a large bowl, combine the ground turkey, cooked brown rice, onion, garlic, oregano, thyme, red pepper flakes (if using), salt, and pepper. Mix well.

4. Place about 1/4 cup of the turkey mixture onto the center of each cabbage leaf. Fold the sides of the leaf over the filling, then roll up tightly.

5. Arrange the stuffed cabbage rolls seam•side down in a baking dish.

6. In a medium bowl, mix together the tomato sauce, diced tomatoes, and lemon juice. Pour the sauce over the stuffed cabbage rolls.

7. Cover the baking dish and bake at 375°F for 45•55 minutes, until the cabbage is tender and the filling is cooked through. Serve the stuffed cabbage rolls warm, with the tomato sauce spooned over the top.

This recipe is an excellent choice for the Galveston Diet, as it features lean ground turkey, fiber•rich brown rice, and nutrient•dense cabbage. The tomato sauce provides antioxidants, while the lemon juice adds a bright, tangy flavor. This dish is low in calories and carbs, making it a satisfying and healthy option for women during menopause.

76. Broccoli and Quinoa Salad

Ingredients:

- 1 cup uncooked quinoa, rinsed
- 2 cups low·sodium vegetable broth
- 4 cups broccoli florets, chopped
- 1/2 cup diced red onion
- 1/2 cup diced cucumber
- 1/4 cup chopped fresh parsley
- 2 tbsp olive oil
- 2 tbsp apple cider vinegar
- 1 tbsp Dijon mustard
- 1 tsp honey
- 1/4 tsp salt
- 1/4 tsp black pepper

Instructions:

1. In a medium saucepan, combine the quinoa and vegetable broth. Bring to a boil, then reduce heat to low, cover and simmer for 15·20 minutes, until quinoa is cooked through. Fluff with a fork and let cool.

2. In a large bowl, combine the cooked quinoa, chopped broccoli, diced red onion, diced cucumber, and chopped parsley.

3. In a small bowl, whisk together the olive oil, apple cider vinegar, Dijon mustard, honey, salt, and pepper.

4. Pour the dressing over the quinoa and broccoli salad and toss gently to coat.

5. Refrigerate the salad for at least 30 minutes to allow the flavors to meld.

6. Serve chilled or at room temperature.

This broccoli and quinoa salad is a perfect choice for the Galveston Diet. It's packed with fiber, protein, and antioxidants from the quinoa, broccoli, and other vegetables. The olive oil and apple cider vinegar dressing provides healthy fats and a tangy flavor. This salad is low in calories and carbs, making it a nutritious and satisfying option for women during menopause.

77. Baked Cod with Mediterranean Salsa

Ingredients:

For the Mediterranean Salsa:
• 1 cup diced tomatoes
• 1/2 cup diced cucumber
• 1/4 cup diced red onion
• 2 tbsp chopped fresh parsley
• 1 tbsp chopped fresh basil
• 1 tbsp olive oil
• 1 tbsp red wine vinegar
• 1 garlic clove, minced
• 1/4 tsp salt
• 1/4 tsp black pepper

For the Baked Cod:
• 4 (6 oz) cod fillets
• 1 tbsp olive oil
• 1 tsp dried oregano
• 1/2 tsp garlic powder
• 1/4 tsp salt
• 1/4 tsp black pepper

Instructions:

1. Preheat oven to 400°F. Line a baking sheet with parchment paper.

2. Make the Mediterranean salsa: In a medium bowl, combine the diced tomatoes, cucumber, red onion, parsley, basil, olive oil, vinegar, garlic, salt, and pepper. Stir to mix well and set aside.

3. Pat the cod fillets dry and place them on the prepared baking sheet. Brush the tops of the fillets with the olive oil and sprinkle with the oregano, garlic powder, salt, and pepper.

4. Bake the cod for 12•15 minutes, until it flakes easily with a fork.

5. Serve the baked cod immediately, topped with the Mediterranean salsa.

This recipe is an excellent choice for the Galveston Diet, as it features heart•healthy cod, fresh vegetables, and anti•inflammatory herbs and spices. The Mediterranean salsa adds a bright, flavorful topping to the baked cod. This dish is low in calories and carbs, while providing lean protein, healthy fats, and essential nutrients that are beneficial for women during menopause.

78. Caprese Stuffed Portobello Mushrooms

Ingredients:

• 4 large portobello mushroom caps, stems removed
• 2 tbsp olive oil, divided
• 1 cup cherry tomatoes, halved
• 1/2 cup shredded fresh mozzarella cheese
• 1/4 cup chopped fresh basil
• 2 tbsp balsamic glaze
• 1/4 tsp salt
• 1/4 tsp black pepper

Instructions:

1. Preheat oven to 400°F. Line a baking sheet with parchment paper.

2. Brush the portobello mushroom caps with 1 tbsp of the olive oil and place them cap•side down on the prepared baking sheet.

3. Bake the mushrooms for 10•12 minutes, until they start to soften.

4. In a small bowl, combine the halved cherry tomatoes, mozzarella cheese, chopped basil, the remaining 1 tbsp olive oil, balsamic glaze, salt, and pepper. Stir to mix well.

5. Spoon the caprese filling evenly into the baked portobello mushroom caps.

6. Return the stuffed mushrooms to the oven and bake for an additional 8•10 minutes, until the cheese is melted and the mushrooms are tender.

7. Serve the caprese stuffed portobello mushrooms warm.

This recipe is a great option for the Galveston Diet, as it features nutrient•dense portobello mushrooms, fresh tomatoes, mozzarella cheese, and basil. The balsamic glaze adds a touch of sweetness. This dish is low in carbs and calories, while providing healthy fats, antioxidants, and anti•inflammatory benefits that are beneficial for women during menopause.

79. Tofu and Vegetable Curry

Ingredients:

- 1 block (14 oz) extra•firm tofu, cubed
- 2 tbsp coconut oil
- 1 onion, diced
- 3 cloves garlic, minced
- 1 tbsp grated fresh ginger
- 2 tsp curry powder
- 1 tsp ground cumin
- 1/2 tsp ground turmeric
- 1/4 tsp cayenne pepper (optional)
- 1 cup diced bell peppers
- 1 cup diced zucchini
- 1 cup diced cauliflower florets
- 1 (13.5 oz) can full•fat coconut milk
- 1 cup low•sodium vegetable broth
- 2 tbsp lime juice
- Salt and pepper to taste
- Chopped fresh cilantro for garnish

Instructions:

1. In a large skillet or wok, heat the coconut oil over medium•high heat. Add the cubed tofu and sauté for 5•7 minutes, until lightly browned on all sides. Transfer the tofu to a plate and set aside.

2. In the same skillet, sauté the onion for 3•4 minutes until translucent. Add the garlic and ginger and cook for 1 minute more.

3. Stir in the curry powder, cumin, turmeric, and cayenne (if using). Cook for 1 minute to toast the spices.

4. Add the bell peppers, zucchini, and cauliflower to the skillet. Sauté for 5•7 minutes, until the vegetables start to soften.

5. Pour in the coconut milk and vegetable broth. Bring the mixture to a simmer and let it cook for 10•15 minutes, until the vegetables are tender.

6. Stir the sautéed tofu back into the curry. Add the lime juice and season with salt and pepper to taste.

7. Serve the tofu and vegetable curry warm, garnished with chopped fresh cilantro.

This curry dish is an excellent choice for the Galveston Diet, as it features plant•based protein from the tofu, fiber•rich vegetables, and anti•inflammatory spices. The coconut milk provides healthy fats, while the lime juice adds a bright, tangy flavor. This curry is low in carbs and calories, making it a nutritious and satisfying meal for women during menopause.

80. Grilled Chicken Caesar Salad

Ingredients:

For the Salad:
- 1 head romaine lettuce, chopped
- 1/2 cup shredded Parmesan cheese
- 2 tbsp toasted sliced almonds
- 2 tbsp lemon juice
- 2 tbsp olive oil
- 1 tsp Dijon mustard
- 1 garlic clove, minced
- 1/4 tsp salt
- 1/4 tsp black pepper

For the Chicken:
- 4 boneless, skinless chicken breasts
- 1 tbsp olive oil
- 1 tsp garlic powder
- 1/2 tsp dried oregano
- 1/4 tsp salt
- 1/4 tsp black pepper

Instructions:

1. Preheat grill or grill pan to medium·high heat.

2. In a small bowl, combine the olive oil, garlic powder, oregano, salt, and pepper. Rub the mixture all over the chicken breasts.

3. Grill the chicken for 5·7 minutes per side, until cooked through. Let rest for 5 minutes, then slice or chop the chicken.

4. In a large salad bowl, combine the chopped romaine lettuce, shredded Parmesan, and toasted almonds.

5. In a small bowl, whisk together the lemon juice, olive oil, Dijon mustard, garlic, salt, and pepper to make the dressing.

6. Add the grilled chicken to the salad and drizzle the dressing over the top. Toss gently to coat.

7. Serve the grilled chicken Caesar salad immediately.

This salad is a great option for the Galveston Diet, as it features lean protein from the grilled chicken, healthy fats from the olive oil and almonds, and fiber·rich romaine lettuce. The Parmesan cheese and Dijon dressing add flavor without too many carbs. This dish is low in calories and carbs, making it a nutritious and satisfying meal for women during menopause.

81. Mediterranean Stuffed Bell Peppers

Ingredients:

- 4 large bell peppers, halved lengthwise and seeds removed
- 1 lb ground turkey
- 1 cup cooked quinoa
- 1 cup diced tomatoes
- 1/2 cup crumbled feta cheese
- 1/4 cup chopped fresh parsley
- 2 cloves garlic, minced
- 1 tsp dried oregano
- 1/4 tsp red pepper flakes (optional)
- Salt and pepper to taste
- 1/4 cup grated Parmesan cheese

Instructions:

1. Preheat oven to 375°F. Arrange the bell pepper halves in a baking dish.

2. In a large bowl, combine the ground turkey, cooked quinoa, diced tomatoes, feta cheese, parsley, garlic, oregano, red pepper flakes (if using), salt, and pepper. Mix well.

3. Spoon the turkey and quinoa mixture evenly into the bell pepper halves.

4. Sprinkle the tops of the stuffed peppers with the grated Parmesan cheese.

5. Bake for 30•35 minutes, until the peppers are tender and the filling is hot.

6. Serve the Mediterranean stuffed bell peppers warm.

This recipe is an excellent choice for the Galveston Diet, as it features lean protein from the ground turkey, fiber•rich quinoa, and nutrient•dense bell peppers. The feta cheese, tomatoes, and Mediterranean herbs and spices add flavor and anti•inflammatory benefits. This dish is low in carbs and calories, making it a satisfying and healthy option for women during menopause.

82. Spicy Thai Coconut Soup with Shrimp

Ingredients:

- 1 tbsp coconut oil
- 1 onion, diced
- 3 cloves garlic, minced
- 1 tbsp grated fresh ginger
- 1•2 tsp red curry paste (depending on desired spice level)
- 4 cups low•sodium chicken or vegetable broth
- 1 (13.5 oz) can full•fat coconut milk
- 1 lb peeled and deveined shrimp
- 2 cups sliced mushrooms
- 1 cup sliced baby bok choy
- 2 tbsp fish sauce
- 1 tbsp lime juice
- 1/4 cup chopped fresh cilantro
- Salt and pepper to taste

Instructions:

1. In a large pot or Dutch oven, heat the coconut oil over medium heat. Add the diced onion and sauté for 3•4 minutes until translucent.

2. Stir in the minced garlic, grated ginger, and red curry paste. Cook for 1 minute, until fragrant.

3. Pour in the broth and coconut milk. Bring the soup to a simmer.

4. Add the shrimp, sliced mushrooms, and sliced bok choy. Simmer for 5•7 minutes, until the shrimp are cooked through and the vegetables are tender.

5. Stir in the fish sauce and lime juice. Season with salt and pepper to taste.

6. Remove from heat and stir in the chopped fresh cilantro.

7. Serve the spicy Thai coconut soup with shrimp hot.

This soup is an excellent choice for the Galveston Diet, as it features lean protein from the shrimp, healthy fats from the coconut milk, and a variety of anti•inflammatory vegetables and herbs. The red curry paste provides a spicy kick, while the lime juice and cilantro add freshness. This dish is low in carbs and calories, making it a nutritious and satisfying meal for women during menopause.

83. Veggie and Chickpea Quinoa Bowl

Ingredients:

- 1 cup uncooked quinoa, rinsed
- 2 cups low•sodium vegetable broth
- 1 (15 oz) can chickpeas, rinsed and drained
- 1 cup diced zucchini
- 1 cup diced bell pepper
- 1/2 cup diced red onion
- 2 cups baby spinach
- 2 tbsp olive oil
- 2 tbsp lemon juice
- 1 tsp ground cumin
- 1/2 tsp garlic powder
- 1/4 tsp salt
- 1/4 tsp black pepper
- 2 tbsp crumbled feta cheese (optional)
- Chopped fresh parsley for garnish

Instructions:

1. In a medium saucepan, combine the quinoa and vegetable broth. Bring to a boil, then reduce heat to low, cover and simmer for 15•20 minutes, until quinoa is cooked through. Fluff with a fork and set aside.

2. In a large bowl, combine the cooked quinoa, chickpeas, diced zucchini, bell pepper, and red onion.

3. In a small bowl, whisk together the olive oil, lemon juice, cumin, garlic powder, salt, and pepper.

4. Pour the dressing over the quinoa and vegetable mixture and toss gently to coat.

5. Stir in the baby spinach until wilted.

6. Serve the veggie and chickpea quinoa bowl warm or chilled, topped with crumbled feta cheese (if using) and chopped fresh parsley.

This quinoa bowl is an excellent choice for the Galveston Diet, as it is packed with fiber, protein, and a variety of nutrient•dense vegetables. The chickpeas provide plant•based protein, while the quinoa, olive oil, and vegetables offer anti•inflammatory benefits. This dish is low in calories and carbs, making it a satisfying and healthy option for women during menopause.

84. Turkey and Sweet Potato Hash

Ingredients:

- 1 lb ground turkey
- 2 medium sweet potatoes, peeled and diced
- 1 onion, diced
- 2 cloves garlic, minced
- 1 tsp smoked paprika
- 1 tsp dried thyme
- 1/4 tsp cayenne pepper (optional)
- Salt and pepper to taste
- 2 tbsp olive oil
- 2 cups baby spinach
- 2 eggs (optional)

Instructions:

1. In a large skillet, cook the ground turkey over medium•high heat, breaking it up with a wooden spoon, until browned and cooked through, about 5•7 minutes. Transfer the cooked turkey to a plate and set aside.

2. In the same skillet, heat the olive oil over medium heat. Add the diced sweet potatoes and sauté for 5•7 minutes, until they start to soften.

3. Stir in the diced onion and minced garlic. Cook for 3•4 minutes, until the onion is translucent.

4. Add the cooked turkey back to the skillet. Season with the smoked paprika, dried thyme, cayenne pepper (if using), salt, and pepper. Stir to combine.

5. Reduce heat to low and let the turkey and sweet potato hash cook for 10•15 minutes, stirring occasionally, until the sweet potatoes are tender.

6. Stir in the baby spinach and cook for 1•2 minutes, until the spinach is wilted.

7. Serve the turkey and sweet potato hash warm, optionally topped with a fried or poached egg.

This hash is an excellent choice for the Galveston Diet, as it features lean protein from the ground turkey, fiber•rich sweet potatoes, and nutrient•dense spinach. The spices add anti•inflammatory benefits. This dish is low in carbs and calories, making it a satisfying and healthy meal for women during menopause.

85. Quinoa and Kale Stuffed Tomatoes

Ingredients:

- 4 large tomatoes
- 1 cup cooked quinoa
- 1 cup chopped kale, stems removed
- 1/4 cup crumbled feta cheese
- 2 tbsp chopped fresh basil
- 1 tbsp olive oil
- 1 garlic clove, minced
- 1/4 tsp salt
- 1/4 tsp black pepper

Instructions:

1. Preheat oven to 375°F. Slice the tops off the tomatoes and scoop out the insides, leaving a 1/4•inch shell. Finely chop the tomato insides.

2. In a medium bowl, combine the chopped tomato insides, cooked quinoa, chopped kale, feta cheese, basil, olive oil, garlic, salt, and pepper. Stir to mix well.

3. Stuff the quinoa and kale mixture evenly into the tomato shells.

4. Place the stuffed tomatoes in a baking dish. Bake for 20•25 minutes, until the tomatoes are softened and the filling is hot.

5. Serve the quinoa and kale stuffed tomatoes warm.

This recipe is an excellent choice for the Galveston Diet, as it features nutrient•dense ingredients like quinoa, kale, and tomatoes. The feta cheese adds a creamy, tangy flavor, while the fresh basil provides anti•inflammatory benefits. This dish is low in carbs and calories, making it a satisfying and healthy option for women during menopause.

The combination of plant•based protein, fiber, and antioxidants in this recipe makes it a great choice for the Galveston Diet. The stuffed tomatoes are both delicious and nutritious.

86. Lemon Dill Baked Cod

Ingredients:

- 4 (6 oz) cod fillets
- 2 tbsp olive oil
- 2 tbsp lemon juice
- 2 tbsp chopped fresh dill
- 2 cloves garlic, minced
- 1/2 tsp salt
- 1/4 tsp black pepper

Instructions:

1. Preheat oven to 400°F. Line a baking sheet with parchment paper.

2. In a small bowl, whisk together the olive oil, lemon juice, chopped dill, minced garlic, salt, and pepper.

3. Place the cod fillets on the prepared baking sheet. Drizzle the lemon dill sauce over the top of the fish, making sure to coat all sides.

4. Bake for 12•15 minutes, until the cod is opaque and flakes easily with a fork.

5. Serve the lemon dill baked cod immediately, garnished with additional fresh dill if desired.

This recipe is an excellent choice for the Galveston Diet, as it features heart•healthy cod, which is a lean protein source. The lemon and dill provide bright, fresh flavors, while the olive oil adds healthy fats. This dish is low in carbs and calories, making it a nutritious and satisfying meal for women during menopause.

The combination of omega•3 fatty acids from the cod, anti•inflammatory properties of the dill, and the antioxidant benefits of the lemon make this a great option for the Galveston Diet. It's a simple yet flavorful way to enjoy a delicious and healthy seafood dish.

87. Veggie and Lentil Stir•Fry

Ingredients:

• 1 cup dry brown or green lentils, rinsed
• 3 cups low•sodium vegetable broth
• 2 tbsp sesame oil
• 1 onion, sliced
• 3 cloves garlic, minced
• 1 inch fresh ginger, grated
• 1 red bell pepper, sliced
• 2 cups broccoli florets
• 1 cup sliced mushrooms
• 2 cups baby spinach
• 2 tbsp low•sodium soy sauce or tamari
• 1 tbsp rice vinegar
• 1 tsp sesame seeds
• Salt and pepper to taste

Instructions:

1. In a medium saucepan, combine the lentils and vegetable broth. Bring to a boil, then reduce heat and simmer for 15•20 minutes, until lentils are tender. Drain and set aside.

2. In a large skillet or wok, heat the sesame oil over medium•high heat. Add the sliced onion and sauté for 3•4 minutes until translucent.

3. Stir in the minced garlic and grated ginger. Cook for 1 minute, until fragrant.

4. Add the sliced red bell pepper, broccoli florets, and mushrooms. Stir•fry for 5•7 minutes, until the vegetables are tender•crisp.

5. Add the cooked lentils, baby spinach, soy sauce, and rice vinegar. Toss everything together until the spinach is wilted.

6. Remove from heat and sprinkle with sesame seeds. Season with salt and pepper to taste. Serve the veggie and lentil stir•fry warm.

This stir•fry is an excellent choice for the Galveston Diet, as it is packed with fiber, protein, and a variety of nutrient•dense vegetables. The lentils provide plant•based protein, while the vegetables and sesame oil offer anti•inflammatory benefits. This dish is low in carbs and calories, making it a satisfying and healthy option for women during menopause.

88. Cauliflower Steak with Chimichurri Sauce

Ingredients:

For the Cauliflower Steaks:
• 1 large head of cauliflower, cut into 1•inch thick slices
• 2 tbsp olive oil
• 1 tsp garlic powder
• 1/2 tsp paprika
• Salt and pepper to taste

For the Chimichurri Sauce:
• 1 cup packed fresh parsley leaves
• 1/2 cup packed fresh cilantro leaves
• 3 cloves garlic
• 2 tbsp red wine vinegar
• 1 tbsp olive oil
• 1 tsp dried oregano
• 1/4 tsp red pepper flakes
• 1/4 tsp salt
• 1/4 tsp black pepper

Instructions:

1. Preheat oven to 400°F. Line a baking sheet with parchment paper.

2. In a large bowl, toss the cauliflower slices with the 2 tbsp olive oil, garlic powder, paprika, salt, and pepper until evenly coated.

3. Arrange the cauliflower slices in a single layer on the prepared baking sheet.

4. Roast for 20•25 minutes, flipping halfway, until the cauliflower is tender and lightly browned.

5. While the cauliflower is roasting, make the chimichurri sauce. In a food processor, combine the parsley, cilantro, garlic, red wine vinegar, 1 tbsp olive oil, oregano, red pepper flakes, salt, and pepper. Pulse until a coarse sauce forms.

6. Serve the roasted cauliflower steaks warm, drizzled with the chimichurri sauce.

This recipe is a great option for the Galveston Diet, as it features nutrient•dense cauliflower and a flavorful, antioxidant•rich chimichurri sauce. The olive oil and herbs provide healthy fats and anti•inflammatory benefits. This dish is low in carbs and calories, making it a satisfying and nutritious meal for women during menopause.

89. Greek Lemon Potatoes

Ingredients:

- 2 lbs Yukon Gold potatoes, peeled and cut into 1•inch cubes
- 1/4 cup olive oil
- 1/4 cup fresh lemon juice
- 3 cloves garlic, minced
- 1 tsp dried oregano
- 1/2 tsp salt
- 1/4 tsp black pepper
- 1/4 cup crumbled feta cheese (optional)
- Chopped fresh parsley for garnish

Instructions:

1. Preheat oven to 400°F. Line a large baking sheet with parchment paper.

2. In a large bowl, combine the cubed potatoes, olive oil, lemon juice, minced garlic, dried oregano, salt, and pepper. Toss to coat the potatoes evenly.

3. Spread the seasoned potato cubes in a single layer on the prepared baking sheet.

4. Roast for 30•35 minutes, flipping the potatoes halfway, until they are tender and lightly browned.

5. Remove the potatoes from the oven and transfer to a serving dish.

6. If desired, sprinkle the roasted potatoes with the crumbled feta cheese.

7. Garnish with chopped fresh parsley before serving.

These Greek lemon potatoes are a great option for the Galveston Diet. The Yukon Gold potatoes provide complex carbohydrates, while the olive oil, lemon, and herbs add healthy fats and anti•inflammatory properties. The optional feta cheese provides a creamy, tangy flavor. This dish is relatively low in calories and carbs, making it a nutritious and satisfying side for women during menopause.

The bright, zesty flavors of the lemon and oregano complement the roasted potatoes perfectly. This recipe is a simple yet delicious way to enjoy a Mediterranean•inspired potato dish.

90. Salmon Salad with Dill Dressing

Ingredients:

For the Salmon Salad:
- 1 lb wild•caught salmon fillets
- 1 tbsp olive oil
- 1/4 tsp salt
- 1/4 tsp black pepper
- 5 cups mixed greens
- 1 cup cherry tomatoes, halved
- 1/2 cup sliced cucumber
- 2 tbsp chopped fresh dill

For the Dill Dressing:
- 1/4 cup olive oil
- 2 tbsp white wine vinegar
- 2 tbsp chopped fresh dill
- 1 tbsp Dijon mustard
- 1 tbsp lemon juice
- 1 garlic clove, minced
- 1/4 tsp salt
- 1/4 tsp black pepper

Instructions:

1. Preheat oven to 400°F. Line a baking sheet with parchment paper.

2. Place the salmon fillets on the prepared baking sheet. Brush the top of the salmon with the 1 tbsp olive oil and season with salt and pepper.

3. Bake the salmon for 12•15 minutes, until it flakes easily with a fork. Let cool slightly, then break the salmon into large flakes.

4. In a large salad bowl, combine the mixed greens, cherry tomatoes, sliced cucumber, and chopped fresh dill.

5. Make the dill dressing: In a small bowl, whisk together the 1/4 cup olive oil, white wine vinegar, 2 tbsp chopped dill, Dijon mustard, lemon juice, minced garlic, salt, and pepper.

6. Add the flaked salmon to the salad and drizzle the dill dressing over the top. Toss gently to coat. Serve the salmon salad immediately.

This salmon salad is an excellent choice for the Galveston Diet, as it features heart•healthy wild•caught salmon, nutrient•dense greens and vegetables, and a flavorful dill dressing. The healthy fats from the salmon and olive oil, along with the anti•inflammatory properties of the dill, make this a nutritious and satisfying meal for women during menopause.

91. Ratatouille Stuffed Bell Peppers

Ingredients:

• 4 large bell peppers (any color)
• 1 tablespoon olive oil
• 1 onion, diced
• 3 cloves garlic, minced
• 1 medium zucchini, diced
• 1 medium eggplant, diced
• 1 can (14.5 oz) diced tomatoes
• 2 tablespoons tomato paste
• 1 teaspoon dried oregano
• 1 teaspoon dried basil
• Salt and pepper to taste
• 1/2 cup shredded mozzarella cheese

Instructions:

1. Preheat oven to 375°F. Cut the tops off the bell peppers and remove the seeds and membranes. Place the peppers in a baking dish.

2. In a large skillet, heat the olive oil over medium heat. Add the onion and garlic and cook for 2•3 minutes until fragrant.

3. Add the zucchini and eggplant to the skillet. Cook for 5•7 minutes, stirring occasionally, until the vegetables are tender.

4. Stir in the diced tomatoes, tomato paste, oregano, and basil. Season with salt and pepper to taste.

5. Spoon the ratatouille mixture into the hollowed out bell peppers. Top each pepper with about 2 tablespoons of shredded mozzarella cheese.

6. Bake for 25•30 minutes, until the peppers are tender and the cheese is melted and bubbly.

7. Serve hot. Enjoy!

92. Blackened Shrimp Tacos with Mango Salsa

Ingredients:

For the Mango Salsa:
• 1 ripe mango, diced
• 1/2 red onion, finely chopped
• 1 jalapeño, seeded and finely chopped
• 1/4 cup chopped cilantro
• Juice of 1 lime
• Salt and pepper to taste

For the Blackened Shrimp:
• 1 lb large shrimp, peeled and deveined
• 2 tbsp blackening seasoning (or make your own blend of chili powder, cumin, garlic powder, paprika, salt, and pepper)
• 1 tbsp olive oil

For the Tacos:
• 8•10 small corn or flour tortillas
• Shredded cabbage or lettuce
• Lime wedges for serving

Instructions:

1. Make the mango salsa: In a medium bowl, combine the diced mango, red onion, jalapeño, cilantro, and lime juice. Season with salt and pepper to taste. Refrigerate until ready to serve.

2. Pat the shrimp dry and toss with the blackening seasoning until evenly coated.

3. Heat the olive oil in a large skillet over high heat. Add the seasoned shrimp and cook for 2•3 minutes per side, until charred and cooked through.

4. Warm the tortillas according to package instructions.

5. To assemble the tacos, place a few pieces of blackened shrimp in each tortilla. Top with a spoonful of mango salsa and some shredded cabbage or lettuce.

6. Serve the tacos immediately with lime wedges on the side.

Enjoy your Blackened Shrimp Tacos with the fresh and flavorful mango salsa!

93. Veggie and Quinoa Stuffed Peppers

Ingredients:

- 6 bell peppers (any color)
- 1 cup uncooked quinoa, rinsed
- 2 cups vegetable or chicken broth
- 1 tablespoon olive oil
- 1 onion, diced
- 2 cloves garlic, minced
- 1 cup diced zucchini
- 1 cup diced mushrooms
- 1 (15 oz) can diced tomatoes
- 1 teaspoon dried oregano
- 1/2 teaspoon dried basil
- Salt and pepper to taste
- 1/2 cup shredded mozzarella cheese

Instructions:

1. Preheat oven to 375°F. Cut the tops off the bell peppers and remove the seeds and membranes. Place the peppers in a baking dish.

2. In a medium saucepan, combine the quinoa and broth. Bring to a boil, then reduce heat and simmer for 15•20 minutes, until quinoa is cooked through. Fluff with a fork.

3. In a large skillet, heat the olive oil over medium heat. Add the onion and garlic and cook for 2•3 minutes until fragrant.

4. Add the zucchini and mushrooms to the skillet. Cook for 5•7 minutes, stirring occasionally, until the vegetables are tender.

5. Stir in the diced tomatoes, oregano, basil, salt and pepper. Cook for 2•3 minutes more.

6. Remove the skillet from heat and stir in the cooked quinoa.

7. Spoon the quinoa•veggie mixture into the hollowed out bell peppers, packing it in tightly.

8. Top each stuffed pepper with about 1•2 tablespoons of shredded mozzarella cheese.

9. Bake for 25•30 minutes, until the peppers are tender and the cheese is melted. Serve hot. Enjoy!

94. Greek Turkey Meatballs with Tzatziki Sauce

Ingredients:

For the Meatballs:
• 1 lb ground turkey
• 1/4 cup panko breadcrumbs
• 1 egg
• 2 cloves garlic, minced
• 2 tbsp chopped fresh parsley
• 1 tsp dried oregano
• 1/2 tsp salt
• 1/4 tsp black pepper

For the Tzatziki Sauce:
• 1 cup plain Greek yogurt
• 1 cucumber, peeled, seeded and grated
• 2 cloves garlic, minced
• 1 tbsp chopped fresh dill
• 1 tbsp lemon juice
• 1/4 tsp salt

Instructions:
1. Preheat oven to 400°F. Line a baking sheet with parchment paper.

2. In a large bowl, combine all the meatball ingredients and mix well until fully incorporated. Roll the mixture into 1•inch meatballs and place them on the prepared baking sheet.

3. Bake for 18•20 minutes, until the meatballs are cooked through.

4. While the meatballs are baking, make the tzatziki sauce. In a medium bowl, mix together the yogurt, grated cucumber, garlic, dill, lemon juice and salt. Refrigerate until ready to serve.

5. Serve the warm meatballs with the tzatziki sauce on the side. Garnish with extra chopped parsley if desired.

This recipe is perfect for the Galveston Diet during menopause. The turkey meatballs are a lean protein source, and the tzatziki sauce provides healthy fats from the Greek yogurt. The vegetables and herbs also offer beneficial nutrients. Enjoy!

95. Lentil and Vegetable Soup

Ingredients:

- 1 tbsp olive oil
- 1 onion, diced
- 3 cloves garlic, minced
- 2 carrots, peeled and diced
- 2 celery stalks, diced
- 1 cup green or brown lentils, rinsed
- 6 cups low•sodium vegetable or chicken broth
- 1 (14.5 oz) can diced tomatoes
- 2 tsp dried thyme
- 1 tsp dried oregano
- Salt and pepper to taste
- 2 cups chopped kale or spinach
- Juice of 1 lemon

Instructions:

1. In a large pot or Dutch oven, heat the olive oil over medium heat. Add the onion and garlic and cook for 2•3 minutes until fragrant.

2. Add the carrots and celery to the pot. Cook for 5 minutes, stirring occasionally, until the vegetables start to soften.

3. Stir in the lentils, broth, diced tomatoes, thyme, oregano, and season with salt and pepper to taste.

4. Bring the soup to a boil, then reduce heat and let it simmer for 20•25 minutes, until the lentils are tender.

5. Add the chopped kale or spinach and lemon juice. Cook for 5 more minutes until the greens are wilted.

6. Taste and adjust seasonings as needed.

7. Serve the lentil and vegetable soup hot. Garnish with extra lemon wedges if desired.

This soup is packed with fiber, protein, and nutrients from the lentils, vegetables, and greens. It's a perfect comforting and nourishing meal for the Galveston Diet during menopause. Enjoy!

96. Lemon Herb Grilled Salmon

Ingredients:

- 4 (6 oz) salmon fillets
- 2 tbsp olive oil
- 2 tbsp lemon juice
- 2 tsp dried oregano
- 1 tsp dried basil
- 1 tsp garlic powder
- 1/2 tsp salt
- 1/4 tsp black pepper

Instructions:

1. In a shallow baking dish or resealable plastic bag, combine the olive oil, lemon juice, oregano, basil, garlic powder, salt, and pepper. Add the salmon fillets and turn to coat both sides evenly with the marinade. Cover and refrigerate for 30 minutes to 1 hour.

2. Preheat grill to medium•high heat.

3. Remove the salmon from the marinade and discard any remaining marinade.

4. Grill the salmon fillets for 4•6 minutes per side, or until the fish flakes easily with a fork and reaches an internal temperature of 145°F.

5. Transfer the grilled salmon to a serving platter. Serve immediately, garnished with lemon wedges if desired.

The lemon and herb marinade adds bright, fresh flavors to the salmon. Grilling the salmon gives it a nice char and smoky taste. This is a simple yet delicious way to prepare salmon that's perfect for a healthy meal.

Enjoy your Lemon Herb Grilled Salmon!

97. Portobello Mushroom Fajitas

Ingredients:

- 4 large portobello mushroom caps, sliced
- 1 red bell pepper, sliced
- 1 yellow onion, sliced
- 2 tbsp olive oil
- 2 tsp chili powder
- 1 tsp cumin
- 1 tsp garlic powder
- 1/2 tsp smoked paprika
- Salt and pepper to taste
- 8•10 small flour or corn tortillas, warmed
- Toppings: guacamole, salsa, shredded lettuce, sour cream, etc.

Instructions:

1. In a large skillet or grill pan, heat the olive oil over medium•high heat.

2. Add the sliced portobello mushrooms, bell pepper, and onion. Sprinkle with the chili powder, cumin, garlic powder, smoked paprika, salt and pepper.

3. Cook the vegetables, stirring occasionally, for 8•10 minutes until they are tender and slightly charred.

4. Remove the skillet from heat.

5. To assemble the fajitas, place some of the portobello mushroom and vegetable mixture into the center of a warm tortilla.

6. Top with desired toppings like guacamole, salsa, shredded lettuce, sour cream, etc.

7. Fold the tortilla over the filling and enjoy!

The meaty portobello mushrooms make a delicious vegetarian protein option for these fajitas. The spices and charred vegetables add tons of flavor. Customize the toppings to your liking. Serve with rice, beans, or a fresh salad for a complete meal.

Enjoy your Portobello Mushroom Fajitas!

98. Baked Chicken with Lemon and Garlic

Ingredients:

- 4 boneless, skinless chicken breasts
- 2 tbsp olive oil
- 3 cloves garlic, minced
- 2 tbsp fresh lemon juice
- 1 tsp lemon zest
- 1 tsp dried oregano
- 1/2 tsp salt
- 1/4 tsp black pepper
- 1 lemon, sliced

Instructions:

1. Preheat oven to 400°F. Lightly grease a baking dish or line with parchment paper.

2. In a small bowl, whisk together the olive oil, garlic, lemon juice, lemon zest, oregano, salt, and pepper.

3. Place the chicken breasts in the prepared baking dish. Pour the lemon•garlic mixture over the chicken, making sure to coat all sides.

4. Arrange the lemon slices around the chicken.

5. Bake for 25•30 minutes, until the chicken is cooked through and reaches an internal temperature of 165°F.

6. Remove the chicken from the oven and let it rest for 5 minutes before serving.

7. Serve the baked chicken warm, drizzled with any pan juices. Garnish with extra lemon slices if desired.

This Baked Chicken with Lemon and Garlic is a perfect option for the Galveston Diet during menopause. The lean protein from the chicken, along with the healthy fats from the olive oil, provide essential nutrients. The lemon and garlic add bright, flavorful accents without the need for heavy sauces or seasonings.

Pair this chicken with roasted vegetables or a fresh salad for a complete and nourishing meal. Enjoy!

99. Veggie and Chickpea Buddha Bowl

Ingredients:

- 1 cup cooked quinoa or brown rice
- 1 (15 oz) can chickpeas, rinsed and drained
- 1 cup roasted sweet potato cubes
- 1 cup roasted broccoli florets
- 1 cup shredded kale or spinach
- 1/2 avocado, sliced
- 2 tbsp toasted pumpkin seeds
- 2 tbsp tahini dressing (recipe below)

For the Tahini Dressing:
- 2 tbsp tahini
- 2 tbsp lemon juice
- 1 tbsp water
- 1 tsp honey
- 1 garlic clove, minced
- Salt and pepper to taste

Instructions:

1. Prepare the tahini dressing by whisking together all the dressing ingredients in a small bowl. Set aside.

2. In a large bowl, layer the cooked quinoa or brown rice, chickpeas, roasted sweet potato, roasted broccoli, and shredded kale or spinach.

3. Top the bowl with sliced avocado and toasted pumpkin seeds.

4. Drizzle the tahini dressing over the top of the bowl.

5. Serve immediately and enjoy!

This Veggie and Chickpea Buddha Bowl is a nutritious and satisfying meal that fits perfectly with the Galveston Diet during menopause. The combination of complex carbs, protein, healthy fats, and fiber·rich vegetables provides sustained energy and supports overall health.

The tahini dressing adds a creamy, nutty flavor that ties all the flavors together. Feel free to customize the vegetables based on your preferences.

100. Grilled Veggie Platter with Hummus

Ingredients:

- 1 zucchini, sliced into 1/2-inch thick rounds
- 1 yellow squash, sliced into 1/2-inch thick rounds
- 1 red bell pepper, cut into 1-inch pieces
- 1 yellow onion, cut into 1-inch wedges
- 8 oz cremini or button mushrooms, halved
- 2 tbsp olive oil
- 1 tsp dried oregano
- 1/2 tsp garlic powder
- Salt and pepper to taste
- 1 cup hummus (store-bought or homemade)
- Lemon wedges for serving

Instructions:

1. Preheat grill or grill pan to medium-high heat.

2. In a large bowl, toss the sliced zucchini, squash, bell pepper, onion, and mushrooms with the olive oil, oregano, garlic powder, salt, and pepper until evenly coated.

3. Arrange the seasoned vegetables in a single layer on the hot grill. Cook for 4-6 minutes per side, or until tender and lightly charred.

4. Transfer the grilled vegetables to a serving platter.

5. Serve the grilled veggie platter with the hummus on the side. Garnish with lemon wedges.

This Grilled Veggie Platter with Hummus is a fantastic option for the Galveston Diet during menopause. The variety of nutrient-dense vegetables provide fiber, vitamins, and minerals. The hummus adds a creamy, protein-rich dip that's full of healthy fats from the tahini and olive oil.

This dish is easy to prepare, visually appealing, and incredibly satisfying. Enjoy it as a main course or as a side to grilled fish or chicken. It's a versatile and wholesome meal that fits perfectly with the Galveston Diet guidelines.

101. Turkey and Kale Stuffed Acorn Squash

Ingredients:

- 2 acorn squash, halved and seeded
- 1 tbsp olive oil
- 1 lb ground turkey
- 1 onion, diced
- 3 cloves garlic, minced
- 2 cups chopped kale
- 1 tsp dried thyme
- 1/2 tsp dried sage
- Salt and pepper to taste
- 1/4 cup grated Parmesan cheese (optional)

Instructions:

1. Preheat oven to 400°F. Place the acorn squash halves cut-side up on a baking sheet. Drizzle with olive oil and season with salt and pepper. Roast for 30-40 minutes, until tender when pierced with a fork.

2. In a large skillet, cook the ground turkey over medium heat, breaking it up with a wooden spoon, until no longer pink, about 5-7 minutes.

3. Add the diced onion and minced garlic to the skillet. Cook for 2-3 minutes until fragrant.

4. Stir in the chopped kale, thyme, sage, salt, and pepper. Cook for 5 more minutes, until the kale is wilted.

5. Remove the roasted acorn squash halves from the oven. Scoop the turkey and kale mixture into the center of each squash half, packing it in tightly.

6. If desired, sprinkle the top of each stuffed squash half with a tablespoon of grated Parmesan cheese.

7. Return the stuffed squash to the oven and bake for an additional 10-15 minutes, until the cheese is melted and the filling is hot. Serve the turkey and kale stuffed acorn squash immediately.

This dish is perfect for the Galveston Diet during menopause. The acorn squash provides complex carbs, fiber, and nutrients, while the turkey and kale offer lean protein and antioxidants. It's a satisfying and nutritious meal that fits the diet's guidelines.

102. Mediterranean Baked Chicken

Ingredients:

- 4 boneless, skinless chicken breasts
- 2 tbsp olive oil
- 2 tbsp lemon juice
- 2 tsp dried oregano
- 1 tsp dried basil
- 3 cloves garlic, minced
- 1/2 tsp salt
- 1/4 tsp black pepper
- 1 cup cherry tomatoes, halved
- 1/2 cup kalamata olives, pitted and halved
- 1/4 cup crumbled feta cheese

Instructions:

1. Preheat oven to 400°F. Lightly grease a baking dish or line with parchment paper.

2. In a shallow bowl, whisk together the olive oil, lemon juice, oregano, basil, garlic, salt, and pepper.

3. Add the chicken breasts to the bowl and turn to coat both sides evenly with the marinade.

4. Arrange the marinated chicken in the prepared baking dish.

5. Scatter the halved cherry tomatoes and kalamata olives around the chicken.

6. Bake for 25•30 minutes, until the chicken is cooked through and reaches an internal temperature of 165°F.

7. Remove the dish from the oven and sprinkle the crumbled feta cheese over the top. Serve the Mediterranean Baked Chicken warm, garnished with extra lemon wedges if desired.

This Mediterranean•inspired baked chicken dish is perfect for the Galveston Diet during menopause. The lean protein from the chicken, healthy fats from the olive oil and olives, and antioxidants from the tomatoes and herbs make it a nutritious and flavorful meal.

The bright, fresh flavors of the lemon, garlic, and Mediterranean herbs complement the chicken beautifully. Serve this with a side of roasted vegetables or a fresh salad for a complete and satisfying Galveston Diet•friendly dinner.

103. Roasted Cauliflower with Tahini Sauce

Ingredients:

For the Roasted Cauliflower:
• 1 head of cauliflower, cut into florets
• 2 tbsp olive oil
• 1 tsp ground cumin
• 1/2 tsp paprika
• Salt and pepper to taste

For the Tahini Sauce:
• 1/4 cup tahini
• 2 tbsp lemon juice
• 1 garlic clove, minced
• 2•3 tbsp water
• Salt and pepper to taste

Instructions:

1. Preheat oven to 400°F. Line a baking sheet with parchment paper.

2. In a large bowl, toss the cauliflower florets with the olive oil, cumin, paprika, salt, and pepper until evenly coated.

3. Spread the seasoned cauliflower in a single layer on the prepared baking sheet.

4. Roast for 20•25 minutes, flipping halfway, until the cauliflower is tender and lightly browned.

5. While the cauliflower is roasting, make the tahini sauce. In a small bowl, whisk together the tahini, lemon juice, garlic, and a pinch of salt and pepper.

6. Add the water 1 tablespoon at a time, whisking continuously, until the sauce reaches a pourable, creamy consistency.

7. Transfer the roasted cauliflower to a serving dish. Drizzle the tahini sauce over the top.

8. Serve the Roasted Cauliflower with Tahini Sauce warm or at room temperature.

This dish is a perfect option for the Galveston Diet during menopause. The roasted cauliflower provides fiber, vitamins, and minerals, while the tahini sauce adds healthy fats and a creamy, nutty flavor.

The combination of the tender, spiced cauliflower and the rich, tangy tahini sauce makes for a delicious and nutritious side dish or vegetarian main course. Enjoy!

104. Shrimp and Vegetable Skewers with Chimichurri

Ingredients:

For the Chimichurri Sauce:
• 1 cup fresh parsley, chopped
• 3 cloves garlic, minced
• 2 tbsp red wine vinegar
• 1 tbsp olive oil
• 1 tsp dried oregano
• 1/4 tsp red pepper flakes
• Salt and pepper to taste

For the Skewers:
• 1 lb large shrimp, peeled and deveined
• 1 zucchini, cut into 1·inch pieces
• 1 red bell pepper, cut into 1·inch pieces
• 1 red onion, cut into 1·inch pieces
• Olive oil for brushing

Instructions:

1. Make the chimichurri sauce: In a small bowl, combine the parsley, garlic, red wine vinegar, olive oil, oregano, and red pepper flakes. Season with salt and pepper to taste. Set aside.

2. Preheat grill or grill pan to medium·high heat.

3. Thread the shrimp, zucchini, bell pepper, and onion onto skewers, alternating the ingredients.

4. Brush the skewers lightly with olive oil on all sides.

5. Grill the skewers for 2·3 minutes per side, until the shrimp are opaque and the vegetables are tender.

6. Transfer the grilled skewers to a serving platter. Drizzle the chimichurri sauce over the top.

7. Serve the Shrimp and Vegetable Skewers with Chimichurri immediately, while hot.

This dish is a perfect option for the Galveston Diet during menopause. The shrimp provide lean protein, while the vegetables offer fiber, vitamins, and minerals. The chimichurri sauce adds a flavorful, herbal punch without the need for heavy dressings or marinades.

The grilled components give this meal a nice smoky, summery flavor. Serve it with a side salad or roasted potatoes for a complete and nourishing Galveston Diet·friendly meal.

Enjoy your Shrimp and Vegetable Skewers with Chimichurri!

105. Greek Orzo Salad

Ingredients:

- 1 cup uncooked orzo pasta
- 1 cup cherry tomatoes, halved
- 1 cucumber, diced
- 1/2 red onion, thinly sliced
- 1 cup crumbled feta cheese
- 1/4 cup kalamata olives, pitted and halved
- 2 tbsp chopped fresh parsley
- 2 tbsp chopped fresh dill
- Juice of 1 lemon
- 2 tbsp olive oil
- 1 tsp red wine vinegar
- 1 tsp dried oregano
- Salt and pepper to taste

Instructions:

1. Cook the orzo according to package instructions. Drain and rinse under cold water to cool completely.

2. In a large bowl, combine the cooked and cooled orzo, cherry tomatoes, cucumber, red onion, feta cheese, olives, parsley, and dill.

3. In a small bowl, whisk together the lemon juice, olive oil, red wine vinegar, oregano, salt, and pepper.

4. Pour the dressing over the orzo salad and toss gently to coat.

5. Cover and refrigerate the Greek Orzo Salad for at least 30 minutes to allow the flavors to meld. Serve chilled or at room temperature. Enjoy!

This Greek Orzo Salad is a refreshing and flavorful dish that's perfect for a light lunch or side. The combination of the chewy orzo, crisp vegetables, briny olives, and tangy feta creates a delicious Mediterranean·inspired salad.

The lemon·oregano dressing ties all the flavors together beautifully. This salad can be made ahead of time and keeps well in the refrigerator for a few days.

Serve the Greek Orzo Salad on its own or alongside grilled chicken, fish, or vegetarian protein for a complete and satisfying meal.

106. Turkey and Spinach Stuffed Mushrooms

Ingredients:

- 12 large mushrooms, stems removed and finely chopped
- 1 tbsp olive oil
- 1/2 lb ground turkey
- 2 cloves garlic, minced
- 1 cup baby spinach, chopped
- 2 tbsp grated Parmesan cheese
- 2 tbsp breadcrumbs
- 1 tsp dried oregano
- Salt and pepper to taste

Instructions:

1. Preheat oven to 375°F. Lightly grease a baking sheet.

2. Remove the stems from the mushrooms and finely chop them.

3. In a skillet, heat the olive oil over medium heat. Add the chopped mushroom stems, ground turkey, and garlic. Cook for 5•7 minutes, breaking up the turkey as it cooks, until the turkey is browned and cooked through.

4. Remove the skillet from heat and stir in the chopped spinach, Parmesan cheese, breadcrumbs, and oregano. Season with salt and pepper to taste.

5. Stuff the mushroom caps evenly with the turkey and spinach mixture, packing it in tightly.

6. Arrange the stuffed mushrooms on the prepared baking sheet.

7. Bake for 15•18 minutes, until the mushrooms are tender and the filling is hot.

8. Serve the Turkey and Spinach Stuffed Mushrooms warm.

These stuffed mushrooms make a great appetizer or light main dish. The combination of savory ground turkey, fresh spinach, and Parmesan creates a delicious filling that complements the earthy mushroom caps.

The breadcrumbs help bind the filling together and add a nice texture. You can adjust the seasonings to your taste, adding more herbs or spices as desired.

107. Quinoa and Vegetable Stir•Fry

Ingredients:

• 1 cup uncooked quinoa, rinsed
• 2 cups low•sodium vegetable or chicken broth
• 1 tbsp sesame oil
• 2 cloves garlic, minced
• 1 inch piece fresh ginger, grated
• 1 red bell pepper, sliced
• 1 cup broccoli florets
• 1 cup sliced mushrooms
• 1 cup snow peas or snap peas
• 2 tbsp low•sodium soy sauce or tamari
• 1 tbsp rice vinegar
• 1 tsp sesame seeds (optional)
• Salt and pepper to taste

Instructions:

1. In a medium saucepan, combine the quinoa and broth. Bring to a boil, then reduce heat, cover and simmer for 15•20 minutes, until quinoa is cooked through. Fluff with a fork.

2. In a large skillet or wok, heat the sesame oil over medium•high heat. Add the garlic and ginger and cook for 1 minute until fragrant.

3. Add the sliced bell pepper, broccoli, mushrooms, and snow peas. Stir•fry for 5•7 minutes, until the vegetables are tender•crisp.

4. Stir in the cooked quinoa, soy sauce, and rice vinegar. Toss everything together until well combined.

5. Season the stir•fry with salt and pepper to taste. Serve the Quinoa and Vegetable Stir•Fry hot, garnished with sesame seeds if desired.

This quinoa and veggie stir•fry is a nutritious and flavorful one•dish meal. The quinoa provides complex carbs and protein, while the colorful vegetables offer fiber, vitamins, and minerals.

The Asian•inspired flavors from the soy sauce, ginger, and sesame oil make this dish incredibly tasty. Feel free to swap in any of your favorite stir•fry vegetables.

108. Lemon Garlic Roasted Shrimp

Ingredients:

- 1 lb large shrimp, peeled and deveined
- 2 tbsp olive oil
- 3 cloves garlic, minced
- 1 tbsp lemon juice
- 1 tsp lemon zest
- 1 tsp dried oregano
- 1/2 tsp red pepper flakes (optional)
- Salt and pepper to taste
- Lemon wedges for serving

Instructions:

1. Preheat oven to 400°F. Line a baking sheet with parchment paper.

2. In a large bowl, toss the shrimp with the olive oil, garlic, lemon juice, lemon zest, oregano, and red pepper flakes (if using). Season with salt and pepper.

3. Arrange the seasoned shrimp in a single layer on the prepared baking sheet.

4. Roast for 8•10 minutes, until the shrimp are opaque and cooked through.

5. Remove the roasted shrimp from the oven and transfer to a serving dish.

6. Serve the Lemon Garlic Roasted Shrimp immediately, with lemon wedges on the side for squeezing over the top.

This simple yet flavorful shrimp dish is perfect for a quick and healthy meal. The lemon, garlic, and oregano create a bright, Mediterranean•inspired seasoning that complements the sweet, tender shrimp.

The roasting method cooks the shrimp quickly without drying them out. Serve the Lemon Garlic Roasted Shrimp over a bed of greens, with roasted vegetables, or alongside whole grains like quinoa or brown rice for a complete and balanced meal.

Enjoy this easy and delicious Lemon Garlic Roasted Shrimp!

109. Eggplant and Chickpea Tagine

Ingredients:

- 1 tbsp olive oil
- 1 onion, diced
- 3 cloves garlic, minced
- 1 tsp ground cumin
- 1 tsp ground coriander
- 1 tsp paprika
- 1/2 tsp ground cinnamon
- 1/4 tsp cayenne pepper (optional)

- 1 medium eggplant, cut into 1·inch cubes
- 1 (15 oz) can chickpeas, drained and rinsed
- 1 (14 oz) can diced tomatoes
- 1 cup vegetable or chicken broth
- 2 tbsp chopped fresh parsley
- Salt and pepper to taste
- Cooked couscous or quinoa, for serving

Instructions:

1. In a large pot or Dutch oven, heat the olive oil over medium heat. Add the diced onion and sauté for 3·4 minutes until translucent.

2. Stir in the minced garlic, cumin, coriander, paprika, cinnamon, and cayenne (if using). Cook for 1 minute until fragrant.

3. Add the cubed eggplant, chickpeas, diced tomatoes, and broth. Bring the mixture to a simmer.

4. Reduce heat to medium·low and let the tagine simmer for 20·25 minutes, stirring occasionally, until the eggplant is very tender.

5. Remove from heat and stir in the chopped parsley. Season with salt and pepper to taste.

6. Serve the Eggplant and Chickpea Tagine warm, over a bed of cooked couscous or quinoa.

This Moroccan·inspired tagine is a hearty, vegetarian·friendly dish that's packed with flavor. The combination of eggplant, chickpeas, and aromatic spices creates a comforting and satisfying meal.

The long simmering time allows the flavors to meld together beautifully. Adjust the amount of cayenne pepper to control the heat level.

110. Greek Stuffed Tomatoes

Ingredients:

- 6 medium tomatoes
- 1 cup cooked quinoa
- 1/2 cup crumbled feta cheese
- 1/4 cup chopped fresh parsley
- 2 tbsp chopped fresh dill
- 2 tbsp olive oil
- 1 tbsp lemon juice
- 1 clove garlic, minced
- 1/4 tsp dried oregano
- Salt and pepper to taste

Instructions:

1. Preheat oven to 375°F. Slice the tops off the tomatoes and scoop out the insides, leaving a 1/4·inch shell. Finely chop the tomato insides.

2. In a medium bowl, combine the chopped tomato insides, cooked quinoa, feta cheese, parsley, dill, olive oil, lemon juice, garlic, and oregano. Season with salt and pepper.

3. Stuff the tomato shells evenly with the quinoa·feta mixture, packing it in tightly.

4. Place the stuffed tomatoes in a baking dish. Bake for 20·25 minutes, until the tomatoes are tender and the filling is hot.

5. Remove the stuffed tomatoes from the oven and let cool for 5 minutes before serving.

6. Serve the Greek Stuffed Tomatoes warm or at room temperature.

These Greek·inspired stuffed tomatoes make a delicious and healthy appetizer or light main dish. The quinoa filling provides fiber and protein, while the feta, herbs, and lemon add bright, Mediterranean flavors.

The tomato shells act as the perfect vessel for the flavorful stuffing. You can adjust the filling ingredients to your taste, adding more herbs, spices, or even diced vegetables.

Enjoy these Greek Stuffed Tomatoes as part of a balanced meal or as a standalone dish. They're sure to be a crowd·pleasing favorite!

As you reach the end of **"The Galveston Diet Cookbook to Manage Menopause: 100+ Nutrient-Rich Recipes to Support Your Journey,"** it's important to reflect on the incredible strides you've made towards embracing a healthier, more vibrant life during menopause. This cookbook was designed not just to provide you with recipes, but to equip you with the knowledge and tools necessary to navigate this significant life transition with confidence and grace.

The Galveston Diet is more than a temporary eating plan; it's a lifestyle shift that focuses on anti-inflammatory, nutrient-dense foods to support hormonal balance, weight management, and overall well-being. By incorporating these recipes and principles into your daily routine, you have taken a proactive step towards mitigating the common symptoms of menopause, enhancing your energy levels, and improving your quality of life.

We hope that the diverse and delicious recipes in this book have inspired you to experiment in the kitchen and enjoy the process of nourishing your body. From hearty breakfasts to sustain you through the morning, to satisfying dinners that bring your day to a close on a high note, each dish is crafted to support your health and wellness goals.

Beyond the recipes, remember the practical tips and strategies provided throughout the book. Meal planning, mindful eating, and staying informed about the nutritional value of the foods you consume are all integral parts of the Galveston Diet lifestyle. These habits will serve you well beyond menopause, contributing to a sustained sense of vitality and well-being.

Thank you for allowing us to be a part of your journey. Embracing change is never easy, but with the right support and resources, it can be a rewarding and transformative experience. As you continue on your path, may you find joy and satisfaction in the meals you prepare and the vibrant health you cultivate.

Here's to a future filled with health, happiness, and the delicious flavors of the Galveston Diet. Cheers to your continued journey towards wellness and to thriving through menopause and beyond!